AMAZING SPINAL PROTOCOL SECRETS THAT WORK!

Achieving Spinal Health
WITHOUT Drugs or Surgery!

Dr. Alan Khiger

Manufactured & Printed in the United States of America.

ISBN: 9781679975028

Dr. Alan Khiger
Amazing Spine Care

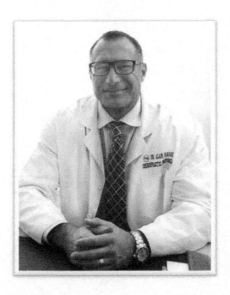

Dr. Alan Khiger is a graduate of Life University, School of Chiropractic Medicine, Atlanta, GA, Licensed Doctor of Chiropractic Medicine in Florida, and has worked in this capacity in personal injury, workers comp and cash practice patients for the past 12 years. Also certified by the American College of Addictionology in Auricular therapy for patients who develop substance abuse disorder, Dr. Khiger's specialties include working with the elderly, children, and new/pregnant mothers.

He has held professional positions in both specialty and general practice chiropractic care, one of his favorite specialties is that of neuro-musculoskeletal disorders.

Dr. Khiger is a healer, and well versed in how to help people find alignment and holistic bodily health. In addition, he fluently speaks three languages: Spanish, Russian, and English.

Learn More: www.AmazingSpineCare.com

Table of Contents

This book contains some of the most advanced technological protocols, combined with traditional chiropractic medicine that had worked amazingly well for me, as well as my patients.

I have been studying spinal conditions for 15 years and have treated over 10,000 patients over my career. My goal was to create the most tactically advanced health care possible; and I can say with confidence that I had achieved my dream. We have come a long way as a society who pioneered inventions and creations that have saved thousands of lives. Some examples would be organ transplants, antibiotics, and MRI machines. Integrating new technologies for the spinal protocols mentioned in this book has raised the standard of Chiropractic Medicine above and beyond our wildest expectations. Because of my research and experience, I felt compelled to share this with the world in need of quality health care.

My fascination with this work continues as I get inspired, and I dedicate this book not only to myself, but my patients as well. My story is never-ending when it comes to spinal conditions. Years ago, I had been suffering from spinal conditions for many years and I continue to suffer as I am involved in the high-impact combat MMA sport. Therefore, I became the personal "doctor to myself" as well as to my patients.

There are currently 88% percent of Americans who are suffering from the chronic disease of neck and back pain. It is currently an epidemic which costing way above the 100-billion-dollar mark. Spinal conditions do not discriminate by age, gender, or race; they will attack anyone and everyone at any point in their lives.

Therefore, being informed by reading this book, you will have an abundance of knowledge; not only understanding these disorders, but also knowing what the optimum choice would be in selecting the right medical help to fight these conditions. The information in this book has not been taught anywhere in the world;

it contains many research studies pertaining to some, but not all, of the conditions at this time.

The market is currently saturated with specialists who claim they have the solutions to your back and neck problems, but unfortunately, it's never going to be a straight cookie-cutter solution. Medicine of any type is not exact science; this is why there are spiritual healers who have helped thousands of patients suffering from various types of illnesses, including the new disease of addiction.

The sickness of various addictions only has a 33% success rate; the 67% failure results in death. This is unlike spinal conditions that have a high favorability of successful outcomes. Mental disorders such as addiction and depression carry a wide range of other related illness which will not produce favorable outcomes in any of the mentioned spinal diseases you will learn about in this book.

Today, patients are more educated than ever before through the use of the internet which has made the job of doctors easier in drawing a line between fact and myth.

The chapters in this book will provide a personal connection to your injury or illness for anyone in your family. This book is not designed to convince you to come and treat your injuries at my clinics in Florida, but to decide based on facts and not mythical stories. You can use www.Spinehealth.com as your reference for verification of some of this material for your own personal information. www.Pubmed.com is another great resource full of databases of researched peer-reviewed articles. I use tools like these to help derive some of the complex conditions my patients present with.

This book guarantees you the success rate of 96% percent in beating your spinal disease, even if you have been suffering for many years!

PRAISE

"Amazing Spine Care is the ONLY place to go! Dr. Plotz, Dr. Khiger, and all of the staff are wonderful, personable people. I was in a car accident and immediately went to the hospital to get myself checked out, waited 2.5 hrs. before being seen and was only given some Motrin for my neck pain and was sent home. I came to Amazing Spine Care and they treated me like a human and not just another patient. They made sure to check all the bells and whistles so that I was cared for by what my specific needs are. Dr. Plotz has amazing healing capabilities, my neck pain and headaches are gone! I will continue to use Amazing Spine Care as my preferred chiropractor, and I would recommend them to anyone!"
— Lacey Shoener

"The staff is great, and the chiropractors are thorough. After a year of chronic neck pain, I was finally able to feel some relief just a few visits."
— Hanna Thompson

"Excellent care, excellent staff! Amazing Spine Care lives up to their name. I highly recommend them. Everyone is super nice, and I always feel amazing after my appointments."
— Rose Ramolete

"Great service, great chiropractor, I highly recommend the very accommodating staff who offer a variety of service. When I started, I was in severe lower back pain after I was assigned a regiment it wasn't permanent, it grew with me healing. I never felt like I came here and wasted time. Decompression machine adjustment exercises and therapeutic messages coupled with a great chiropractor is the key. As said earlier highly recommended."
— Sam Bosque

"These people here are amazing. They treat you good and make you feel like family. They answer all my questions I have. I will always come back."

– Shelby Mann

Chapter 1

Acute Disc Conditions

The acute disc condition occurs when you had aggravated it by lifting something heavy at work, or at home. It can also cause a sudden onset when you travel or just wake up in the morning to go about your day.

The acute disc pain is severely intense, and you will need accommodation from your significant other to help you move around. At that point there no magic pills or drugs that can subdue your pain or provide any kind of relief you are looking for.

The pain has no discrimination for age, gender, or size; it will take you to your knees no matter how tough you are.

The acute disc injury will target 3 regions:

1. Neck
2. Mid-back
3. Low back

Amazing Spine has set a protocol in place for our patients. They will either come in twice a day for three days, or every day for five days. The treatment we typically administer is spinal manipulation of the symptomatic region. We also use spinal decompression set at lower values than ice and electric stem unit to decrease the inflammation in the spine.

I want you to understand that inflammation is the fire that occurs in your body as a result of an injury, and it is the body's response saying, "Please fix me, I am injured!"

Acute disc protocol must be managed with anti-inflammatory medications. Over the Counter meds such as Ibuprofen or Motrin will block the cascade of the inflammation in your blood; you will also want to use ice for 15 min every hour if possible.

Chapter 2

Chronic Disc Protocol

The Chronic Disc Protocol is another disc condition that occurs in your spine but is there for a longer time. The chronic disc protocol can be a tolerated pain for the first episode when someone is thinking that it will go away on its own and masking the pain with meds or pain injections. It can also occur as a result of unhealed trauma in the spine.

The Chronic Disc Protocol has a very high rate of surgical interventions due to low-level knowledge and lack of research available in the field. Most chronic disc conditions are caused by disc herniations, disc bulges, disc protrusions/extrusions, and various nerve impingements.

The chronic disc conditions will produce numbness and tingling in the arms if it is found in the neck. It can also cause numbness and/or tingling in the legs if it is found in the lumbar (low back) spine.

The diagnostic tool of an MRI or X-ray is a preferable choice for Neuro/Ortho surgeons as well as chiropractors. The chronic disc can produce many false positive pain distribution factors such as:

- Radiating pain in the buttock
- Shooting pain into the mid back
- Belt distribution pain in the low back

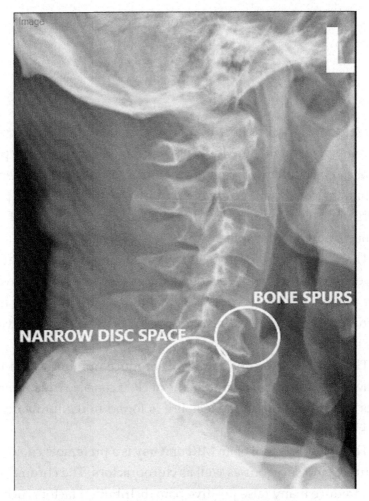

Figure 1. X-ray of the patient with chronic neck pain, radiating down the arm.

Some patients describe it as a shooting needle-like pain. The pain can also be caused by a deteriorated disc in the spine particularly in the geriatric population. In either instance we have managed these conditions with a 96% success rate and have been able to reverse every surgical decision for our patients!

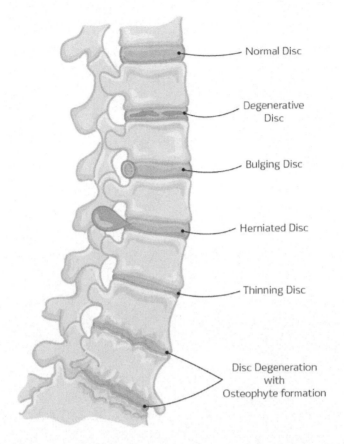

Normal Disc

Degenerative Disc

Bulging Disc

Herniated Disc

Thinning Disc

Disc Degeneration with Osteophyte formation

Figure 2. Common disc problems include degenerative disc disease.

The patients are treated with spinal manipulation, spinal decompression, functional rehabilitation, and an ice/heat electric stem and laser unit. The frequency of the plan varies on the length of suffering, diagnostic imaging and the age of the patient.

The protocol can always be altered as the patient's symptoms improve or worsening. If the patient was feeling good with a gradual reduction of pain and then the symptoms flared up and got worse; then the protocol gets to be intense and the patient can be seen every day or two times a day as warranted. The worsening can be caused by being overweight, an unhealthy lifestyle or overuse such as re-injury or various kinds of trauma.

Chapter 3

Super Max Protocol

The Super Max Protocol is one of my favorites but is used very rarely.

This protocol is used on patients who are obese, extremely overweight, who have no strength in their legs or arms, or who have excruciating pain in their neck and back when drugs or injections have failed them.

This type of protocol can also be utilized for patients who have been under our care for a while, but got worse due to an additional injury, over-working for many hours, or some sort of trauma.

The patient comes in for treatment twice a day for a maximum of three days straight. The management of care is:

- Spinal manipulation
- Spinal decompression
- Ice
- Electro Therapy (electro muscle stem unit)
- Laser

The patient is forbidden to use any functional rehab until day two of their treatment. The patient then goes back to his or her original protocols for treatment of their damaged discs in their spine.

The estimated improvement from the Super Max Protocol is between 70-80% which is very favorable for the patient. The patient must then be placed on a regular treatment schedule to obtain the 96% improvement we desire for them.

Herniated disc   Spinal decompression

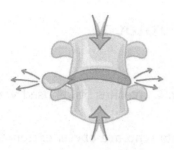 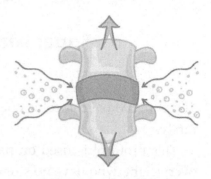

Pressure in the disc is so great that
a tear occurs in the disc wall leading
to back pain (numbness an tingling)

A reduction of pressure inside the disc
(decompression) aids in drawing nutrients,
oxygen and moisture back into the disc

**Figure 3. Disc herniation showed on the left image.
Absorption of the fluid back into a disc space thus
relieving pressure of the nerve showed on the right.**

Chapter 4

Sciatica

Sciatica is a symptomatic term associated with a pinched nerve in the leg. The sciatic nerve is the longest nerve in the body, and it originates in the lumber spine, goes through the piriformis muscle and then runs through the back of the leg.

The sciatic nerve pain will cause numbness in the leg, loss of sensation, pain in the buttock, and atrophy (muscle shrinkage) in the muscle. If left untreated it may produce a condition known as the "foot drop" (partial paralysis of the nerve in the lower extremity).

The sciatic nerve is a secondary component of low back pain. In fact, most of the time, the patient will not have any low back pain, even if you hit them with a hammer! The reason for this is due to a pain receptor which is called the nociceptor which carries pain into the brain for interpretation. The nociceptors are usually cause by trauma to the region via accident or slip and fall.

Therefore, one should not be fooled. It should be treated it as a dual diagnosis of back pain where it came from, and what is targets. The exam will definitely produce weakness in the leg and decreased reflexes. Management of sciatic pain is:

- Spinal manipulation of the lumbar spine
- Spinal decompression
- Passive and active (doctor involved or patient) stretching of the piriformis muscle.

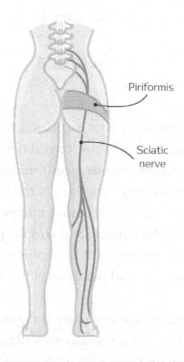

Piriformis

Sciatic
nerve

Figure 4. Piriformis entrapment of sciatic nerve.

The stretching of the piriformis can be achieved with the patient face-down or upright, depending on the doctor's preference.
The weakness in sciatic nerve distribution will always be caused
by the pinched nerve in the back and signal the piriformis for
severe pain when sitting.

The success rate at our clinics is favorable, producing 98% recovery in our patients.

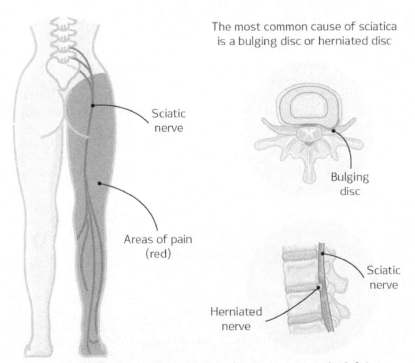

The most common cause of sciatica is a bulging disc or herniated disc

Sciatic nerve

Bulging disc

Areas of pain (red)

Sciatic nerve

Herniated nerve

Figure 5. Sciatic nerve trapped inside the disc space on the left image, the pattern of the nerve distribution on the right.

Chapter 5

Rehab Protocol

As a former patient, I went through four years of spinal rehabilitation of my leg and spine after an injury I had in Odessa, Ukraine when I was only six years old from falling from the tree.

The exercise protocol became mandatory at my offices. I love building them, implementing them, and watching my patients benefit from them!

The injured disc will cause injury to the nerve, as well as the muscle and any competent doctor who performs a muscle test on the patient's arms or legs will observe their arm or leg drop with resistance. The reason for this is that the pinched nerve fully controls the function of the muscle, and once that nerve is under pressure, just like a balloon under pressure, it will pop, spill water, and cause pressure on that spinal nerve. When this happens, the long-term injury immediately shrinks the muscle by a process called atrophy and strength and productivity diminish.

That is why physical therapists are trained to perform exercises to strengthen the weak and injured muscles on the patients who fail balance tests, grip tests and coordination. The Functional Rehab Protocols are specific, so if you are suffering from low back pain, you will be performing exercises to strengthen all the muscles around your waist to help you regain stability and control of that injured area.

If you are suffering from neck pain, the muscles around it will need to be strengthened for support and function of your neck. Occasionally you see people wearing a neck brace around their neck after certain automobile injuries. The reason for this is, when whiplash occurs, the cervical spine is susceptible to injuries, and varies fractures can occur at the atlas bone that holds the occiput (the head) together.

At that point, wearing a brace is recommended. However, when you are wearing a brace without a fracture, you are weakening your neck muscles and lose the support of your disc and nerve.

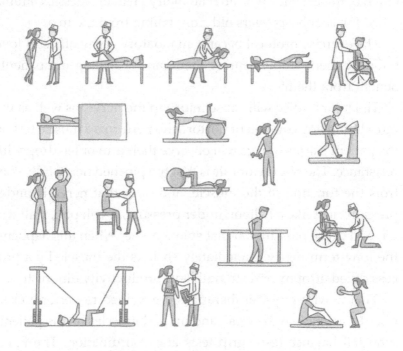

Figure 6. Exercise and functional rehabilitation is the most important part of the therapy, the pain is secondary to function.

This is why it's critical to strengthen the muscles to achieve the maximum support possible in your spine so you can improve function and heal faster.

In sports we see a lot of athletes get hurt on the field and immediately after they are placed on the bike, go through stretches, or use ice to reduce swelling. These are all common practices in rehabilitation of the injured or damaged tissues that require physiological or mechanical healing.

Chapter 6

Shoulder Protocol (traumatic/arthritic)

The shoulder is an interesting joint due to the fact that it moves in many different directions. Up, down, back, side and diagonally. There are baseball pitchers who injure their shoulder during the game from aggressive throwing, and they are out of commission no less than a year. Why do you think that is?

You guessed it right.

The shoulder has 18 muscles that control its movement and there are also ligaments and tendons that support it. I am not going to go over all of the anatomical structures, but rather talk about the conditions that we treat in our office that are effective and have 99% success rate.

The first common condition is the rotator cuff injury where the muscles of the shoulder girdle get damaged due to overuse at work or working out. This type of condition would be classified as traumatic. The patient is going to have restricted range of motion by not being able to lift the arm above 90 degrees in the direction of the head. If they attempt to move it higher, they will experience severe pain in their shoulder.

The treatment protocol is spinal manipulation of the neck and shoulder then cold laser with the rehab exercises. Patients will come in three times a week for two weeks, then gradually be reduced to twice a week for three weeks to achieve 98% recovery.

Another common condition we see at our office is "frozen shoulder" which happens to be an arthritic condition in nature.

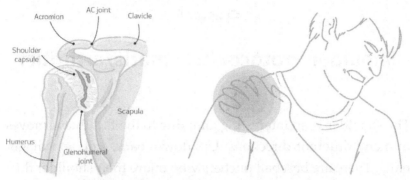

Figure 7. Frozen shoulder presentation of a typical patient who suffered early trauma or overuse.

The patient will experience excruciating pain in their shoulder with the inability of lifting their arm. This typically attacks women, from what I have seen in practice.

The scar tissue builds around the shoulder socket and stiffens the arm with pain and loss of movement. The success rate is 80% with patients who let it go for a long time, but 98% with patients who came to see us earlier.

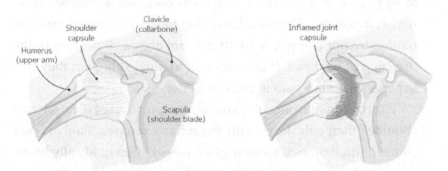

Figure 8. Images of traumatic shoulder pain in the left and inflamed shoulder joint with arthritis.

The number of visits varies from fifteen to twenty-six, depending on severity. This condition is probably the one with the most variation on recovery versus anything else in the spine.

The treatment we implement is spinal manipulation of the patient's neck, then the shoulder with three different maneuvers mobilizing the movement with laser and shoulder functional therapy to stretch out the damaged tissues.

Shoulder Impingement

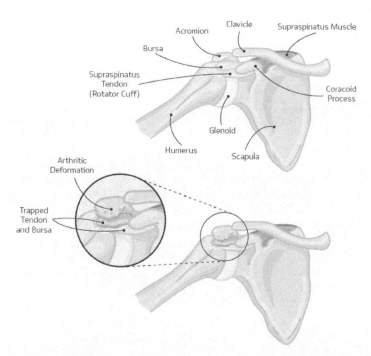

Figure 9. Additional joints in the shoulder that can generate pain manageable with the same protocol.

Chapter 7

Surgical Protocol

This happens to be another one of my favorite topics due to the fact our job is to minimize surgeries and avoid costly mistakes that are irreversible during the surgery.

I personally am not against surgeries and would never talk someone out of surgery if they need one. But the reality is this, even neurosurgeons and orthopedists now talk their own patients out of surgery themselves due to high failure rates that have been estimated close to 70%. A great source of that would be www. Spinehealth.com where surgeons themselves encourage patients to seek second opinions and ask doctors if they would operate on themselves if they had a similar condition!

In my experience, I had reversed thousands of surgical recommendations from the time I practiced in San Diego with the use of Spinal Decompression which is currently discussed as a tactical protocol in this book. Surgery is always advised as the last option for the patient when all else fails. Some side effects of surgery can include infections, permanent paralysis, and chronic pain associated from the scar tissue.

It is an undeniable fact that chiropractic would not have been offered as an option on the same level as the neurosurgeons and orthopedists if it were not for the invention of the Spinal Decompression machine. As a new school chiropractor who implements this treatment on a daily basis against chronic disc conditions, we have more medical practitioners who have more trust and confidence in our work than ever due to the safety and effectiveness of this great invention.

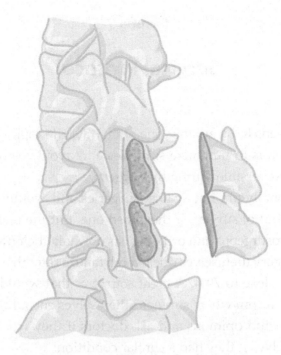

Figure 10. Surgical Lumbar laminectomy

The surgical interventions work greatly on patients with torn tissues. It is like doing an upgrade on a building that has been demolished. When that happens, you would need to lay a new foundation with new materials. The surgeons use materials such as screws in your spine, metal plates, and cutting through your bones with the procedures such as a Laminectomy, discectomy, or spinal fusions to relieve the pressure on the pinched nerve that is causing your pain.

What we do and they do is the same approach of relieving pain on the nerve, but we do it with the use of hands and spinal decompression; they use the knife and scissors to get to the removal of disc material that is leaking and obstructing your nerve. This is no different than when a woman gives birth and the OB-GYN uses forceps to pull on the baby's head which can cause structural damage; or they use the hands to gently extract the head from the womb.

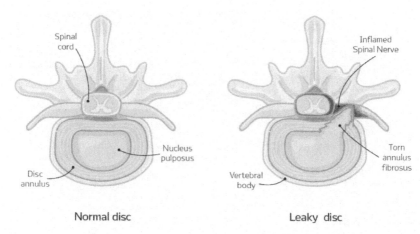

Figure 11. Another demonstration of a leaky disc putting pressure on the nerve producing pain.

Chapter 8

Post Surgical Protocols

This chapter is based on work that I performed for a patient for his low back after the Laminectomy was performed on his lumbar spine. He was and elderly Asian man who came to me with the complaint of neck pain, and had been recommended surgery for his neck due to a herniated disc.

He underwent 20 successful spinal decompression treatments with spinal manipulation of his neck and was 98% better. My curiosity was why he came to my practice? He said that he came because he had surgery on his back and still had pain and numbness in his left leg. He came in wondering if there would be any chance, I could take a look at it and see if it could be fixed.

After I looked at your X-ray's and see what type of surgery was done, it showed he had the Laminectomy done on his L4-S1. I immediately I said without hesitation "I will take your case!" My rationale was that he had some disc space left and preserved allowing me to decompress and manipulate it to relieve the extra pressure placed on the nerve. His pain generator in his back that was producing pain was the disc and the facet joint at L5/S1. The post surgical fusion of L4/L5 did not produce the nerve pain into the leg or follow its pattern of distribution into the foot.

The patient was then placed on a protocol of three times a week for three weeks consisting of chiropractic adjustments to the pelvis and lumbar spine decompression. I also performed Functional Rehab with a gradual reduction to twice a week for three weeks. The patient was 97% better and was grateful for the treatment plan put together for him that saved him from yet another surgery!

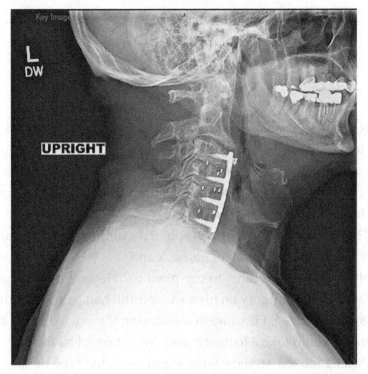

Figure 12. Surgical fusion of the damaged discs in the neck.

Another post-surgical case was a woman in San Diego I treated who presented with sever localized neck pain after a surgical fusion of C5/6. Currently there are 90% of surgeries are performed in this location because the most amount of movement that that joint produces like moving the head up and down. The X-ray showed screws in her Cervical Spine, but we were able to perform spinal manipulation of the regions above and below to release the pressure on the nerves through the degenerated discs. We also utilized spinal decompression of her Cervical spine with low force pressure pull.

The patient also underwent Functional Rehab of her neck and upper back to strengthen the musculature and was placed on a protocol of three visits a week for three weeks with gradual reduction to two visits a week for three weeks to get to a 95% improvement!

Chapter 9

Knee Protocol

Patients that come to our office with knee pain is quite common. The population that is affected with the knee pain most, is just about anyone who works standing on their feet for a long period of time or is involved in any sport. Another example of common knee pain would be osteoarthritis. This could include hairdressers, bank tellers, nurses, construction workers, waitresses and overweight patients.

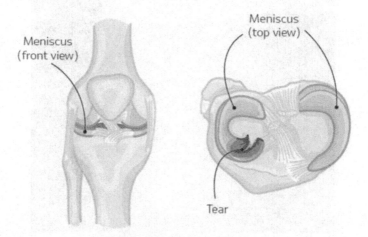

Figure 13. Meniscl tear in the knee.

The knee is a compensatory mechanism that bears the load of the body which starts to put pressure on the Menisci that is located on each side of the knee. The purpose of that Menisci is to protect your knee from a shocking mechanism just like the shocks on the car which prevents the car from slamming to the ground.

The material of the Menisci in your knee is made up of the same type of watery-like substance of the discs in your vertebral spine. Once it is confirmed that there is meniscus pain, we pre-scribe a protocol of three times a week for two weeks and then move to twice a week for three weeks. We begin by first adjusting the Pelvic Joint along with the Lumbar Spine Joints to correct the compensatory pain.

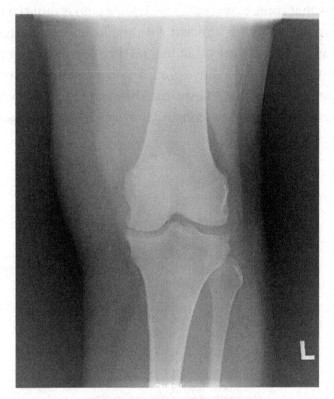

Figure 14. Arthritic knee joint.

Then we adjust the knee joint according to the restriction of movement and we laser out the affected side of the knee by using ice/heat with electric stem, corrective rehab exercises to strengthen the muscles around it along with orthopedic taping to secure the movement of the ligaments to keep the knee from sliding.

We have seen 99% recovery with our patients with these par-ticular disorders!

Chapter 10

Pelvic Protocol

The pelvis is the most important part of the body due to the fact that it is the foundation that allows you to walk and sit. Also, the pelvis plays a major role in women delivering babies. The pelvis will control all of your neurological connections in your spine all the way to the brain.

There is still not enough research done to prove how all of the neurology fits into place, and most orthopedists and neurosurgeons will agree. But what we do know is that pelvic conditions are very common and produce 98% of your low back pain.

When someone suffers from low back pain, the pelvis is the compensatory body part that picks up the weight-bearing comfortable position for the patient to avoid putting extra pressure on the damaged disc. The pelvis is composed of four bony structures: Ilium, Ischium, Sacrum, and Coccyx. It produces four points of pain arising out of its joint position. It will cause pain from the Sacra Iliac joint that connects the Ileum and Sacrum in the back of the pelvis in an area called the "Mickey Mouse Ears."(see the pic below)

The ears have two levels: the upper and the lower level. The upper ear pain will prevent your leg from bending forward. Then the pain coming from the lower "Mickey Mouse Ear" will flair your leg into the side and produce a similar dull pain in your low back. The frontal pain from the groin results from the pubis bone that shifted.

Very rarely I have seen patients with just pelvis issues alone at my office, it is always as a result of the low back pain that is related to herniated or bulged discs.

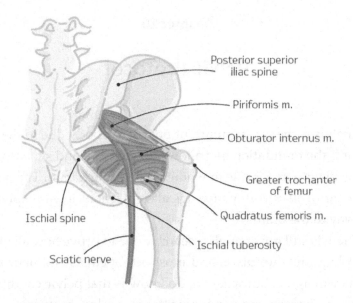

Figure 15. Nerve entrapment located in the pelvic area.

The Pelvic Protocol is rapid, typically a total of 5 visits, due to the fact there are no discs involved like in the spine, and because there is no disc, recovery expected 99% of the time. However, If the spine is involved then the duration is much longer depending on severity.

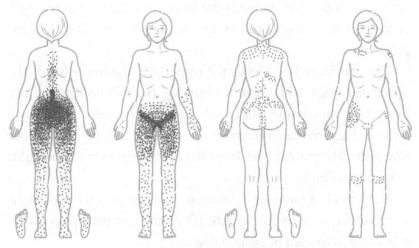

Figure 16. Pelvic pain pattern as a result of sciatic pain which happens 99% of the time.

Chapter 11

Headache Protocol

Patients who come to our offices with headaches are typically tension headaches and migraine which target mostly females than males.

The tension headaches are produced by tight muscles around the neck. These tight muscles will start pulling on the spine as if someone is trying to take your head off. The pressure that is produced in your spine on all the soft tissues by the tight muscles will cause headache pain in your head.

The migraine headaches are caused by abnormal neurological pathways that are associated by nerve toxicity. The nerve toxicity can be caused from the food you eat; for example: excess alcohol, energy drinks (Red Bull), stimulant drugs, or processed food like cheese and marinated products.

The use of medication for relieve of headaches is temporary and will not produce lasting effects. In fact, all of the over-the-counter products contain Acetaminophen which is a toxic pharmacological substance that tends to cause toxicity in the blood stream and may increase your susceptibility to headaches after a prolong use.

The headache relief that we have being using for our patients is very simple and reduces your symptoms by 97% after the first visit! The patient is seated, then the doctor places both hands on the back of the neck muscles. Then the patient pushes into the doctor's palm gently compressed against the patient's head for approximately thirty seconds. The doctor then adjusts the patient's neck to relieve the pressure of the tension headache.

Tupes of headaches

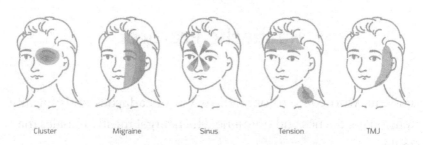

Cluster   Migraine   Sinus   Tension   TMJ

Figure 17. Typical Headache pain pattern.

The chronic tension and migraine headaches are treated three times a week for six weeks utilizing spinal manipulation of the Cervical and Thoracic spine. Ice packs are used to constrict the dilation of the blood-flow into the head that causes headaches, as well as stretching exercises of the short, tight muscles of the neck.

Patients report 90% improvement in their condition. If the improvement is stalled, the patient is encouraged to seek treatment from a medical doctor to co-manage the condition; especially if it is a migraine headache that can be caused by disrupted pathways in the blood or nervous systems.

Chapter 12

Laser Protocol

The cold laser treatments have been a very successful aiding tool in treating muscle strains, ligament strains, tendinitis, neck pain, back pain, and sports injuries. The laser light that is projected out of the tube is a deep penetrating light that shoots 800 nm deep into the damaged cells and produces a healing effect by regenerating new cells through the conversion of physiological processes.

Imagine a woman who is using advanced laser treatment for facial procedures to look young and wrinkle free. This is the same type of technology that utilizes light energy to change the shape of your cells!

Another example would be using the sunlight, which we have a lot of in Florida, to change the color of your skin. Unlike the sunlight that produces damaging UV rays which causes cancer in high doses, this light is absolutely safe to use. We have been using laser light as a helping tool to achieve the maximum improvement in our patients who present with all of the conditions mentioned in this book including arms, wrists, knees, ankles, neck pain, back pain, hip and joint pain.

The success rate is at 98% percent using laser as an extra technology in regenerating new healthy cells!

The laser treatment has also been popular in management of arthritis. Arthritis is a disease that the body develops which loves to attack your joints like the fingers, knees, shoulders and hips. Arthritis destroys the cartilage that is found in your joints; kind of like the oil that is in your engine- if you do not replace the oil in the engine, what is going to happen to your engine? Your engine will burn and then you can throw your car away.

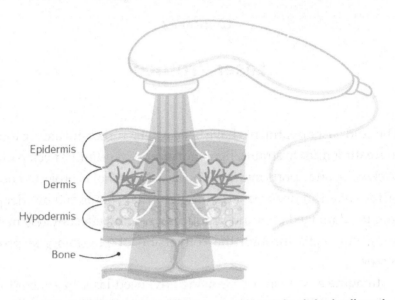

Epidermis

Dermis

Hypodermis

Bone

Figure 18. Typical function of the laser and how it heals bad cells and converts them into new ones.

The same thing is going to happen to you if you do not provide the defenses for your joints necessary for them to function. Patients who currently present with osteoarthritis in the knee take on average fifteen visits to manage. A patient of ours was suffering from severe knee and hip pain associated with arthritis; we placed her on a protocol of three times a week for three weeks with a gradual reduction to twice a week for three weeks. The result was a 75% improvement in function and pain!

The procedures used were spinal manipulation, manipulation of the extremity (knee), laser with heat, stem and functional rehab along with supplementation for rebuilding of cartilage. We advised her to confirm with her primary care physician to avoid any interaction with other meds that she takes. The patient was extremely happy since she battled with this pain for over 20 years. Laser treatments were an important game changer in her condition.

Chapter 13

Tendonitis Protocol

Tendonitis is the inflammation of the tendon that cause severe pain in the shoulder if you are a construction worker, for example, or overusing your arm during repetitive exercises. It is also found in the elbow, shoulders, and ankles with the same symptom and presentation as in the shoulder. The nature of this condition is long-lasting if not taken care of early. A lot of patients will think that this a self-limiting problem and will go away on its own, but this will very rarely happen.

When the tendinitis is hurting longer than expected and you can't use your arm for work, and you are having difficulty feeding your family, then you will need to see a doctor.

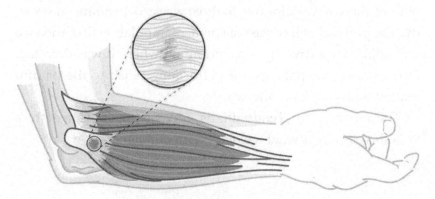

Figure 19. Origin of the tennis elbow pain

Tendonitis conditions are quick to heal, and do not require long-term protocols. However, if they are mixed with another diagnosis, for example, tendinitis of the shoulder from overusing the arm as a construction worker, and rotator cuff strain, then obviously the treatment is extended.

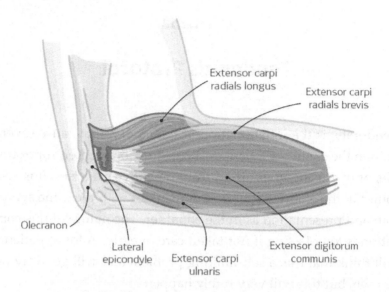

Figure 20. Torn ligament in the same region will produce similar pain as the tennis Elbow

Typically, for straight tendinitis we put patients on a protocol of three times a week for two to three weeks depending on severity. The protocol will consist of spinal manipulation first, then we will adjust the extremity, depending on where it was detected. Furthermore, the patients are performing rehab to the painful tendon with cold laser afterwards.

The recovery for Tendonitis is very favorable. Currently a 98% success rate is what we observe in our clinic.

Chapter 14

TMJ Protocol

The TMJ Protocol happens to be a very interesting one because there are multiple symptoms that currently arise out of the pain associated with the jaw.

Jaw pain can be due to a neurological implication as a result of trigeminal nerve dysfunction or just having their jaw being misplaced as a result of an accident or improper alignment; you can also develop pain due to arthritis of the joint. Remember that arthritis attacks your joints.

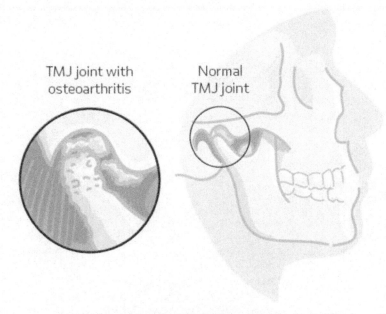

Figure 21. Inflamed joint in the jaw which resembles a typical pattern of the arthritis.

The pain in the jaw can also be mistakenly attributed to false tooth pain which will cause you to visit the dentist, who may tell

you that your jaw is out of alignment. You may begin to feel click-
ing and experiencing slow progression of the symptoms making
it difficult to chew food; this can also lead you to becoming mal-
nourished.

The treatment protocol is very simple, manipulation of the
jaw, exercises for strengthening the TMJ joint, ice, and finally
electric stem therapy. The treatment plan is three times a week
for two weeks, then twice a week for two weeks.

In our clinics, patients report a 98% favorable outcome in pain
reduction and improvement in function such as the ability to
chew food which is very important for survival!

Chapter 15

Scoliosis

Scoliosis is becoming more and more common these days in kids ranging from age 8 to 17 who are complaining of neck and back pain as well as numbness in the legs or arms. In years past, we would typically see symptoms like these in adults who develop them later on in life as the spine degeneration progresses causing multiple injuries to the disc and nerves.

The cause of scoliosis is currently unknown that is why it is called "idiopathic" in medicine (from the word idiot). For some reason scoliosis favors girls more than boys and will impact organs as the patient gets older by increasing the curve of the spine and compressing your lungs and heart.

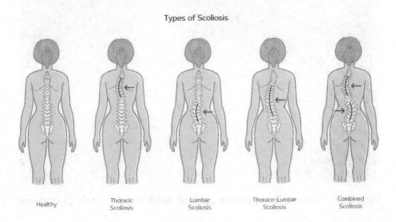

Figure 22. Various scoliotic curvatures that cause spine pain in Children

Scoliosis had three different grades ranging from mild, moderate and severe. The mild range is 5-15 degrees, moderate range is 15-35 degrees, and the severe range is 40 and above. The ones we have been managing most frequently are the ones with mild

to moderate ranges because severe ranges would require a separate technology to manage as well as a separate facility equipped
with specialized machinery.

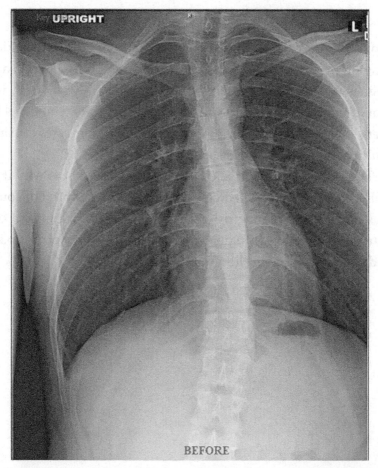

Figure 23. Before. X-ray of the patient with the Scoliotic Curvature.

The tool used to analyze scoliosis conditions is still the good
old X-ray; the images show curvatures of the spines where angles
are measured and assessed. The patient is then instructed to perform stretches five days a week for 30 minutes targeting the con-
vexity of the apex of the spine. The treatment plan can last up to
six months depending on the amount of curve lost. See below.

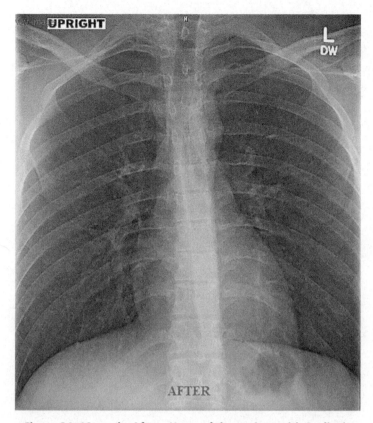

Figure 24. 12 weeks After . X-ray of the patient with Scoliosis

Chapter 16

Vertigo

Benign Positional Vertigo (BPV) is disruption of crystals in your inner ear, that gets popped or busted open like a garbage bag full of trash causing dizziness and loss of balance. Vertigo can also cause Nystagmus which is rapid movement of your eyes.

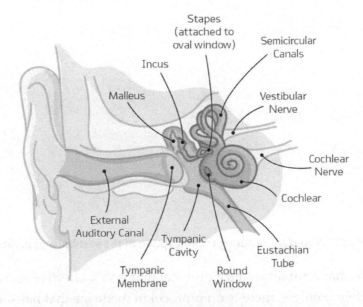

Figure 25. The inner ear anatomy of the vestibular system.

The semicircular canal in your ears is like a convoluted tube that carries water in your sink; its function is simply to maintain the balance of your body. BPV is also very common after car accidents and is sometimes referred to as a Traumatic Brian Injury (TBI).

When someone is diagnosed with Vertigo it is definitely no fun! Also, it is very traumatizing for the patients who must run back to their M.D and/or neurologists for solutions which modern science does not have yet.

The symptoms that I had seen, from my experience operating my practice are devastating. Patients feel like they are falling and have no control of their body in space. They also feel like the room is spinning and they are frightened. The patient absolutely has no control over this situation, but this condition is painless. Imagine someone handcuffed you and threw you under water. How would that feel? You bet, not very nice!

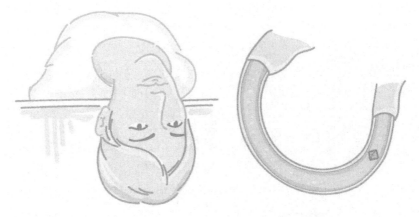

Figure 26. Procedure restoring the disruption of the vestibular apparatus.

We have implemented a protocol that is 99% effective and absolutely painless, there is no protocol in medicine that has more favorable outcome than this one!

The patient first is seated than asked to pinpoint the direction of the dizziness. If the patient turns the head to the right for example and feels, dizzy, the patient is turned over on that side for one minute with their head tilted 45 degrees to the side and back. The patient is then turned over to the opposite side with the same head-tilt for one minute.

Finally, the patient is laid on their back with the same head tilt backward and sideways at 45 degrees for one minute. The head then moved by the doctor to the opposite side at 45 degrees and head-tilt at the same angle and instructed not to tilt their head downward for the entire day. The protocol may be repeated for an additional day, but most patients report full and total recovery after the first treatment!

Chapter 17

Nutritional Protocol

Nutrition is a very broad subject that has many elements and purposes combined to deliver targeted results. There are currently Doctors of Naturopathic Medicine who only use nutrition to heal people with nutritional protocols consisting of herbs, homeopathic remedies, and berries containing therapeutic ingredients.

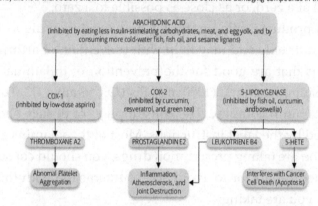

Figure 2. Arachidonic Acid's Destructive Cascade

To better understand the pathways by which arachidonic acid can cause arthritic, carcinogenic, and cardiovascular conditions, the flow chart below shows how arachidonic acid cascades down into damaging compounds in the body.

Figure 27. Sequence pattern of the Arachidonic Acid converting bad foods like Red meat into inflammation.

When someone tells you that "you are what you eat", it is a totally true statement. You can argue with me that there are people who are overweight, not obese,

and they are extremely healthy; there is definitely no argument there. We have seen people who are skinny who are sick, and we see obese people who are sick. Obesity has reached 66% in the United States and was declared a pandemic by the Centers of Disease Control.

Obesity will not only produce spinal problems, but also deadly cardiovascular problems as well. The sugar consumption found in sweets and sugar-coated products will increase the amount of the inflammation in the body that will target the discs on the spine causing pinched nerves in the joints. Dairy products like milk and cottage cheese will cause constipation and bloating and when you have a disc problem, straining in the bathroom trying to pass bowels will not be fun.

Another food product that must be avoided that makes you inflammatory along with the sugar, is red meat. Red meat contains a product called Arachidonic Acid that fuels arthritis in the joints. That is why you see people with "swan lake fingers." Arthritis is not curable, the only thing you can do is keep the arthritis level at a zero, or as close as possible to a zero.

Fish products, chicken, turkey and vegetarian diets are very rich in nutrients and may help with prevention of arthritis. The vitamins that are good for the prevention of inflammation are Magnesium, vitamin C (1000 mg), Fish Oil, vitamin D3, Turmeric, and vitamin B complex. The consumption of dosage should be followed by the label instructions. Most of the vitamins are safe, but if you are taking prescription drugs, you should consult with your medical doctor to avoid any counteraction with the medications you are taking.

Weight loss diets are important to help avoid back pain because is someone is overweight, it will cause more inflammation and extra pressure to be exerted on the spinal disc.

The weight reduction should be started with reduction of sugar first. Secondly the elimination of carbohydrates and starchy foods, such as potatoes and rice must be taken out at dinner prior going to bed. When you sleep all the starchy foods are in a form of sugar that gets converted into fat when you go to sleep. Therefore, protein foods for dinner are the best option for weight management since they do not get converted into complex sugars that turned into fat.

So, the fat is not your enemy, sugar is. The problem with protein diets is that they make you hungry very quickly after eating; therefore, it is recommended that you buy some type of protein replacement shake that has 0 sugars and 0 carbohydrates to satisfy your hunger.

Nutrition is a very broad subject; these are some of the general key points I had outlined here in this chapter. However, if you have medical conditions that will require you to seek medical intervention due to hormonal diseases such as Cushing's, Thyroid disorders, then nutrition doctors who specialize in this field will be a great help for you. There are plenty of these practitioners out there that focus on weight control as well as homeopathic remedies.

Chapter 18

Cane Protocol
(Losing the Walker)

This chapter details a special moment in my career when I first accomplished what seemed to be impossible when I was practicing in Las Vegas.

There was a patient who lived in my building on the same floor, a very pleasant African American women, who used a walker for assistance in getting around. We started talking in the elevator and I was curious and asked if she would mind losing the walker? She replied with a kind smile, "I pray to the Lord every day and I am hoping for some kind of a miracle." I told her since we live in Vegas, miracles happen but not the mirages or illusions acted out during the spectacular shows that the city of lights has to offer!

She agreed to come in for a consultation to my office where I performed an evaluation and told her that it would take a while for her to heal, but we should be able to have her walk and function without the assistance of a walker after approximately two months.

She presented with degenerative disc disease in her low-back, mid-back, and neck with arthritis in her pelvis. She also was recovering from three strokes, so she was screened for safety prior to engaging in treatment for her conditions.

I started manipulating her spine and pelvis, then she was placed on a rehab protocol consisting of strengthening exercises, which worked really well especially after her stroke. After a treatment plan of six weeks of three times a week, she no longer needed a walker!

Her story can be seen on YouTube for anyone who is interested in seeing her incredible journey.

https://youtu.be/bMRBDqPnjfs

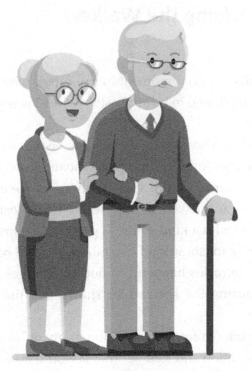

By Iconic Bestiary/Shutterstock.com

**Figure 28. Assisted walkers are commonly used
on patients suffering from chronic low back pain.**

Walkers and canes are used to assist with dysfunction of the spine. If you lost your limb in a war, that is a different story and you will not be needing a walker or a cane, but a prosthetic leg or an arm. If you have done nothing about your spine by seeking medical care, then your spine begins to rot and degenerate like an infected wound that was left untreated and needs to be disinfected. At that point you are dragging your own body in the bag

24 hours a day 7 days a week. The joints in your bones are starting to fill with arthritis and immobility. It's like the old saying: "if you do not use it, you lose it."

Once you have reached permanent loss of function and degeneration, you are going to look like the letter C after developing an ugly hump in your spine that will make you stiff and turn into Frankenstein's monster! You can see those types of people every day, just look at the supermarkets and you will see them riding in the wheelchair, overweight or their head falling down to the floor unable to look in your face.

These are all ignored symptoms of arthrosis joint care that, left untreated, the consequences are unfortunately permanent and irreversible. The objective is to act fast and try to get better and find solutions to the problems.

I have seen in my 12 years of practice, people die a miserable stubborn death because they failed to take care of themselves in this way. I have seen happy people who are always positive overcoming their pain and misery with the treatments of appropriate chiropractic medicine; they are all so grateful and leave positive reviews on our site.

Chapter 19

Misrepresentation of Using Medication for Pain

Drug medications have been used for years going all the way back to 1800's and they carry therapeutic benefits designed to curb the symptoms of pain. There are many different kinds of drugs like psychedelic, tranquilizers, anti-depression, stimulants, and pain-relieving drugs.

Cocaine, for example, is the best anesthetic drug used in oral surgeries by dentists and there are no better or strong drugs out there that can replace it. The nasal recreational use carries a more deadly result by increasing the heart rhythm and damaging cardiovascular system causing cardiac arrest. The pain killer, however, has an adverse effect on the cardiovascular system as they slow your heart rate causing you to die much faster by reducing the amount of blood pumped in your arteries and veins. Both drugs hook on to the receptor to produce a pain-free feeling effect while you are currently on the drug.

Morphine drugs were used in a war after someone had their leg or arm blown off. At that point, the opioid drug must be administered to curb the amount of pain the patient will feel as a result of a torn limb. In today's real world, pain medications are over-prescribed and abused by the patients. The patients make excuses that they are hurt and injured and that they need the opioid to curb their pain. Even hospitals are instructing patients to take 800mg of ibuprofen instead of Oxycodone which contains opioid morphine-based chemicals for pain.

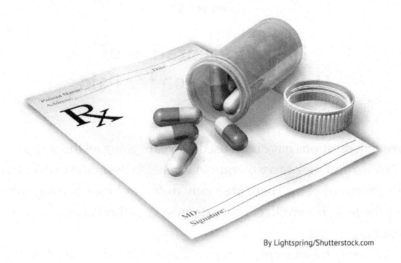

By Lightspring/Shutterstock.com

Figure 29. Narco pain pills often abused by the patients for common treatment of back pain.

The brain has a chemical pathway that leads to the addiction of any substance. Alcohol for example, can turn people into alcoholics which is a condition by far the most dangerous to treat due to the toxicity that the alcohol causes on the tissues. Alcohol destroys all of your organs, not just the liver, which is why you can smell it on someone's breath after they consumed excessive amounts. In moderate amounts, alcohol has been confirmed in studies at 40% prevention of ischemic cardiovascular attacks by breaking down the number of bad cells in the body. The dosage varied from man to women due the body weight and muscle tissue.

I personally do not have anything bad to say as a doctor in regard to the therapeutic drug use versus abuse. I have seen patients die from it in my years of practice from misuse and their health and body not able to tolerate it. There are currently 40,000 people that die every year as a result of medical errors. The reason for this is, as I mentioned earlier, medicine is not an exact science and it's nearly impossible to screen each patient for potential drug overdose or interaction.

Just think how many times you took them and felt fine, then after a while they started making you dizzy, stupid and affected your concentration. That is why each drug must be closely monitored by your physician. If you have reached a maximum therapeutic benefit for the use of a medication, it is time for the reduction or elimination to avoid the danger of the side effect. You do not need to be a doctor to figure this out, it's all common sense.

(Please advise your physician first as I am not a prescribing doctor and can't legally take you off any medication).

Also, a routine blood test should be enforced in making sure the toxins are not destroying your liver or digestive tract.

What I have seen in my practice when it comes to treating elderly people using opioid medications, is that they constantly are complaining of constipation in the stomach. Another symptom I had noted is that getting up from a reclining position to a sitting position produces dizziness. The circulation in the blood is so viscous and heavy that it takes longer for the blood to reach the brain. This is why opioids in the elderly population produce a condition called Orthostatic Hypertension.

Chapter 20

Myths About the
Use of Manual Therapy

Currently only about 8% of the population in the United States are utilizing chiropractic services for their neck pain, back pain, nerve pain, sciatica and various disc conditions. The reason for that is that there is a misinformation about the usage of manual therapy treatment. This type of treatment has been utilized going back as far as the days of Hippocrates. There were no pain medications or pain killers and yet people recovered quickly and spread the word (without internet) throughout the whole world.

Can chiropractic treatment cause pain?

Manual therapy treatment is specific to the defective joint in the body that produces a pinching nerve pain, so why would it hurt if the pain caused by the bone being out place is already hurting?

The bad experiences I had heard that manual therapy was painful is due to a poor ability to diagnose pain in that particular joint. There are currently facilities popping through the United States called "The Joint". I can't make a connection from the name for the life of me, but you can get unlimited Chiropractic visits without the use of X-Ray as long as you pay per month. But, are you willing to risk your neck getting popped without knowing what is internally wrong with you? This is where proper diagnostic tools such as X-ray and MRI must come into play to pinpoint where the problem came from!

For example, if you have neck pain and it produces pain down into your arm and into the first three fingers of your hand, then you know it is related to something pressing on that nerve in your neck. 98% of the time it is a leaky, worn out disc in your

C5/C6 cervical spine pinching the spinal nerve that extends down the arm; or about 2% of the time, it could be a tumor sitting on that nerve and the X-ray or the MRI will show that.

The other myth is that patients think getting a massage will solve their back pain or neck pain issues. The massage will alleviate the pain in the muscle if you have a muscle sprain, but it will not take away the pain related to a disc herniation or disc degeneration.

In fact, we have many patients complaining that the massage makes them feel worse if they presented with pain down the leg or the arm, or if they have been involved in a car accident. The massage has therapeutic benefits for relieving stress, headaches and various types of muscle pain and should be implemented as part of health regimen.

Another myth about chiropractic care is that you have to get treatments forever to feel better. But you must understand that treatment is very specific when it comes to managing these neuromusculoskeletal disorders and consist of specifically designed protocols like I have outlined earlier in these chapters. Will you be seeing a chiropractor for a long time? No. When you want to ensure that you maintain your absolute optimum health, then the answer is yes.

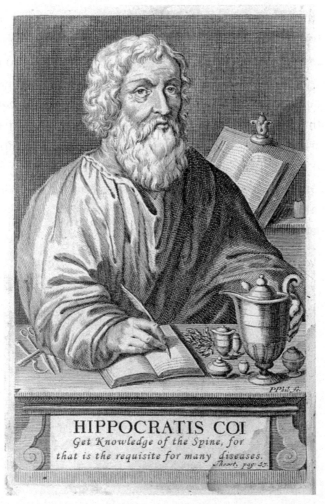

Figure 30. Greeks had created a civilization that still is functional democracy in most of the developed countries. The spine conditions are nothing new as well as the form of treatment.

How many years do you see your family medical practitioner per year? Every year, at least once a month to get a refill on your medications. I worked in a Primary Care clinic and they saw patients, the same type of patients for a period of 20 years. How many times do you visit your dentist a year? So, to jump to a conclusion that you have to see a chiropractor for a long time is absurd.

Another myth is that doctors will tell you never to see a chiropractor. I have heard that many times over and over again. The medical doctors who I talk to encourage patients to go see another chiropractor for the illnesses that they can't manage.

In fact, the medical community has overcome the barrier of separating their treatment and isolating the alternative care. There are currently integrative practices where they implement medical and chiropractic care at the same office. In my experience working with a medical doctor who had the knowledge in Osteopathic medicine has produced wonders for getting my patients better and improving their health.

Chapter 21

Exercise/ Fitness/Working Out

As mentioned previously, I was a very sick kid from my injury. As a result, I lost a lot of muscle tissue to a point where I had to be spoon-fed due to muscle atrophy. My exercise therapist used to always motivate me pushing me to walk and lift weights. My grandfather used to bring pictures of bodybuilders and tell me that one day it is going to be me! Well, in fact, it was during my early 20's I became obsessed with the world of bodybuilding and Arnold Schwarzenegger and I won 1st place in an overall novice competition. Exercise has helped thousands of people with reducing cholesterol, diabetes, and heart disease. Thousands of patients who died from these illnesses, could still possibly be alive today.

A lack of exercise became a public health issue. We currently have the most amount of health clubs and fitness centers with personal trainers, but still the United States is not in first place as the healthiest country in the world. The benefits of exercising include weight loss, improved concentration, more energy, and a reduction in the aging process.

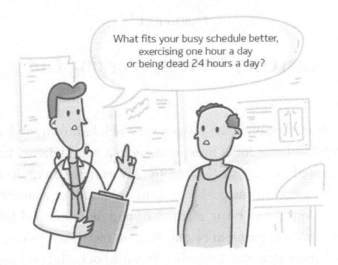

Exercise history goes back as far as Adam and Eve, when you see their portrait both of them look fit. Many Jewish religious congregations are now motivating their attendees to exercise regularly on their own or with a trainer. The reason for this is that many Jewish people suffer with chronic diseases such as arthritis, stroke, high cholesterol and high blood pressure and need to change to a healthier lifestyle.

Heart disease is the number one killer in the United States, the second one is cancer. Exercise reduces the chance of cancer and cardiovascular diseases and there are many studies on Pubmed.com that underline the facts of benefits of exercising.

Exercise can be cardiovascular such as running, walking, swimming, playing tennis, boxing, wrestling etc. Resistance training is great for building your immune cells against viruses that attack them such flu viruses. So, if you are prone to getting sick often and you get your flu shot every year and it's not helping you, then you should immediately engage in consistent resistance training activities.

Many people have a misconception about starting to exercise. They think that if they did not start at an early age then it is already late.

That is a total myth.

You can start exercising at any age, even at 80 years old. There is no age limit on physical activity of any kind. I suggest hiring a trainer in the beginning to help you out with your goals that you set. Without goals you will never succeed. You will stay in one place and will make excuses after setting resolutions at New Year's.

Do not put off living healthy, telling the same lies to yourself every year falling right back where you started. Exercising must be part of your daily routine to achieve success in life and business with health and more endurance.

I can't stress enough the importance of exercising at any age of your life.

Chapter 22

Spiritual Healing

Spiritual healing is an extremely powerful medicine that is very popular in the United States but has not been widely advertised. This type of medicine is very affective in the management of stress, release of toxins, as well as treatment of addictions. Pretty much every drug and alcohol rehab in the country has a spiritual healer that treats addicts, and the insurance pays for all of it.

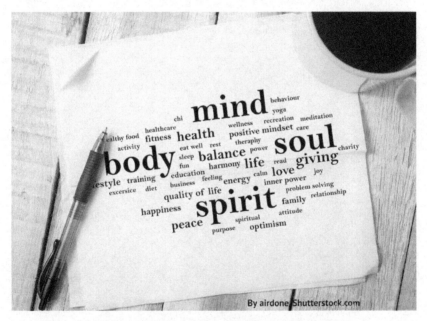

By airdone Shutterstock.com

Figure 32. Spiritual healing does not only have to be Yoga it exists in many different forms.

Spiritual treatment interventions examples are Yoga, Acupuncture, Meditation and Reiki; these remedies will not be effective in treating back and neck pain but will reduce the stress associated with neck and back pain. Many patients have claimed they used these therapies and had benefited from the elimination of pain, but there are no studies that directly proves that this type of treatment produced any favorable results in patients with severe disc conditions or numbness and tingling in the arms and legs.

However, utilizing acupuncture and mindfulness along with chiropractic care and spinal decompression have demonstrated improvement in patients complaining of low back pain. Therefore, utilizing spiritual healing for stress, depression, low immunity, low energy etc. has earned a solid position in the health care arena with proven record in research and management.

Chapter 23

Mental Health and Chronic Pain

There have been a great number of correlations found between mental health and chronic low back pain. Just think when you are faced with stressful situation due to a death in the family, getting fired at your job, getting into a verbal dispute over nothing. (If this has not happened to you yet and you are trying to deny the fact that it affects you, then you are an emotionless human being.)

But those of us who have experienced this, unfortunately it is a part of life. I have known and seen people with chronic low-back pain and neck pain to be depressed, make irrational decisions, and even taking their own life.

We had a Russian patient who had a great, good-looking family who came to this country as immigrants and achieved a level of success in life and business. He was suffering from chronic low back pain for a period of three years and was managed by a medical doctor for pain who prescribed opioid medication for him. One day he turned the gun on himself and committed a suicide. Tragedies like this, have been going on for 300 years where people were killing themselves by suffering from the severe pain that would not respond to remedies or cures.

We don't have to go too far back to remember Dr. Kevorkian who was behind the invention of the "suicide machine" that was killing terminal patients who would rather die than live with pain for their entire life. In reality it can happen to anyone and that is a scary thought.

The longevity of chronic low-back pain or neck pain will produce damaging effects on the mind. The psychomotor response

is part of our physiology in dealing with the neurological stress-
ors. How many times you heard elderly people complain of pain
due to being depressed from cancer or poor nursing home envi-
ronment?

It happens all the time, so it is no myth that mental health is a
contributing factor of your back and neck pain. We treated a 90+
year old patient after I did a speech on spine health at a nearby
nursing home facility. He began coming in for treatments for his
low-back pain and was always preoccupied about how badly the
conditions were at the nursing home facility and how he hated
being there more so than talking about the cause and improvement of his back pain. He wound up dropping from care due to
no transportation available to the office for the treatment and his
kids were too busy working to bring him along.

Just a very sad story all around, what if he had a car and able
to drive? What if he was not living at nursing home and had been
able to drive to treatments like other patients that we have at our
office? You bet the outcome would be different with his recovery
and healthy outcome.

Another similar case was another female elderly patient who
was suffering from chronic low-back pain and neck pain who
was in her late 70's. She came in for treatments at our office and
was complaining of depression and loneliness but was more active than the 90-year-old gentlemen who resided with her at the
same nursing home. We immediately referred her over to coun-
seling and directed her to get involved in meditation and mindfulness. She was treated for depression and made remarkable
recovery as well as improvement in her neck and low back pain.

The last example I would like to cover is a U.S soldier who
was treated for his low-back pain due to an accident. He was diagnosed with a PTSD at the age of 55. Very pleasant African
American fellow and I had great pleasure in working with him.

Not only we were able to get him to a 92% improvement, he also got a job and moved out of the homeless shelter.

Psychological factors will always cause prolonged pain, the treatment must be rendered to both roots of the problem. If one is left without the other the patient will never get better. Please see the cascade model below.

MENTAL HEALTH
— AND —
CHRONIC PAIN

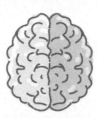

Patients with symptoms of depression are **thee times** more likely to report experiencing chronic physical conditions than the general population

Patients with physical conditions are **twice as likely** to also experience mood or anxiety disorder than the general population

source:
Canadian Mental Health Association

DEPRESSION

Depression is the most common psychological condition associated with chronic pain

source:
American Chiropractic Association

DISABILITY

Chronic pain and depression combined is often associated with preater disability than either depression or chronic pain alone

source:
American Chiropractic Association

In any given year, 1 in 5 patients experiences a mental health problem or illness

Mental illness costs the patients economy more than $50 billion each year

4,000 patients die every year as a result of suicide, most of them were suffering a mental illness

of all approved disability claims in the federal service in 2010 were due to mental health condition

Patients like these must join support groups and become involved or their wellbeing will be in jeopardy. Support group therapy works, they work for alcoholics, women that had miscarriages, veterans returning from war who are disabled, victims of 911 terrorist attacks, and the list goes on and on.

Chapter 24

Carpal Tunnel Syndrome

Carpal tunnel syndrome has been a major factor in wrist pain primarily in women. The disease involves an entrapped nerve in your tunnel in the wrist called the "median nerve." The bones that make up that tunnel are called "carpal". When you have been diagnosed with carpal tunnel syndrome or CTS as they call it, your option according to the internet are splinting and surgery. In this book, we are not talking anyone out of surgery, but why would you do it if you had alternative options? It's like jumping in the fire without looking for routes of escape. I do not know anyone who would willingly do that!

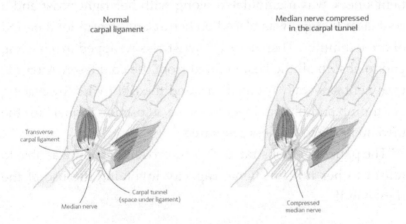

Figure 33.17 Example of how the median nerve gets trapped inside the wrist causing pain

The wrist gets a slightly different holistic approach using manual therapy than that of the neck and wrist. The reason for that is that nerve originates in the neck, branching through the shoulder and into the wrist. Nerve health has to be relieved, always at the root, then the distal entrapment at the wrist becomes a secondary component that must be treated for total fast recovery of pain and symptoms.

One of the main groups susceptible to carpal tunnel, are women as I mentioned before. This is due to the types of jobs that they currently have. It can be a sitting desk posture syndrome that leads to carpal tunnel syndrome by overloading the pressure on the wrist and the muscles of the neck. It can also be a stay-at-home mom who cooks and cleans, and does manual labor raising the kids. The mechanism of injury is the same nerve entrapment arising out of the neck that leads into the wrist causing pressure at the carpal tunnel.

We had a stay-at-home mom one time as a patient who had developed carpal tunnel syndrome. We placed her on a treatment plan consisting of three times a week for three weeks with a gradual reduction to twice a week for three weeks. The patient's neck was manipulated along with her right wrist and a cold laser therapy was placed on her distal forearm for a period of three minutes. Then her right wrist was wrapped in a heating pad to absorb all the heat emitted from the cold laser. After the treatment she was "K-taped" around the right wrist by placing her thumb and pinkie finger to create a "pseudo tunnel" for the median nerve to feel less pressured.

The patient demonstrated 97 % improvement and was able to return to her full functional capacity involving the use of the right hand!

Chapter 25

Ankle/Foot Pain

Foot pain along with ankle sprain are very common conditions we treat at our office. The foot is composed of bones, ligaments, and tendons and there are no discs in the feet. There are many conditions that are associated with pain in the feet such as Achilles tendinitis, arthritis, diabetes, bunions, gout, plantar fasciitis, heel spur, and more. That is why there is a whole medical specialty focused on the treatment of feet which is called podiatry. We are going to discuss the conditions that we see at our office and implementing our new breakthrough protocols in healing them.

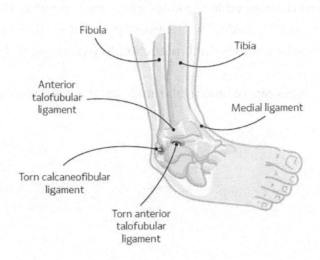

Figure 34. Example of the talofibular sprain in the foot.

The first condition is a sprain of the talofibular ligament that is located one inch from the midline of the foot. The purpose of that structure is moving your feet up, down and side-to-side. As we talked about before, wherever we have the most moveable joint in the body, the amount of wear and tear is greatly increased. Therefore, injuring this ligament during running, walking, and playing sports is a very likely. The pain is felt immediately and lasts a long time due to the elastic property of the structure which is equivalent to a plastic bag in the supermarket. If you over-stretch the plastic bag, is it going to go back, or is it going to stay overstretched? You right it's going to stay overstretched!

The same concept applies to an overstretched ligament due to twisting or bending. The treatment that we provide for ankle sprains consists of the following: First, we adjust the pelvis and the lumbar spine to eliminate any leg inequality. Then we adjust the injured foot via an instrument or hands-on. Then cold laser is placed directly on the talofibular ligament for a period of three minutes. The patient is then placed on an electric stimulation unit with a pack of ice over it for a period of fifteen minutes. Finally, the patient is wrapped in the kinesis tape for support of the liga-ments around the ankle. The treatment plan is three times a week for two weeks with gradual reduction to twice a week for two weeks.

The success rate of healing the ankle sprains are 99% effective!

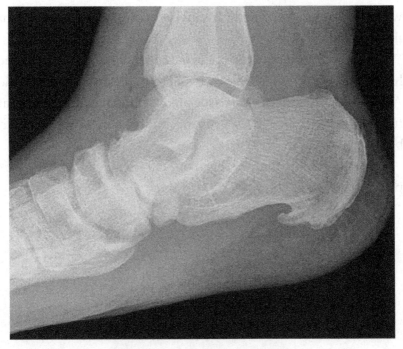

Figure 35. X-ray of the heel spur.

The next common foot pain that we see at our office is heel spur pain. This pain would be felt by the patient at the back of the foot and radiate to the heel and x-ray analysis is best for diagnosing it. The radiological image will show an actual spur attached to the heel of the foot. Once it is confirmed and established, we move on to the treatment portion. First, we adjust the pelvis and the lumbar spine to remove any leg inequality. Then we adjust the foot and the heel to remove any misplacement of the bones there. Then we apply Ultrasound therapy on to the foot for a period of eight minutes to deliver healing properties into the arthrosis tissue. Then we apply heat for a period of ten minutes to recruit red blood cells for additional healing properties due to the fact that heel spur is not an injury, but a self-grown disease. Finally, we wrap the heel up with the Kinesio tape to ease the pressure on the foot. The patient is seen three times a week for three weeks with gradual reduction twice a week for three weeks.

The patient is instructed not to eat red meat while treating the heel spur pain; the reason for this is to block any release of the Arachidonic Acid build up associated with eating red meat that fuels arthritis and causes arthritic buildup in the joints and bones.

The success rate that we see in our clinics managing heel spur pain is 98% effective!

Chapter 26

Elbow Pain

Elbow pain is extremely common at our office and we have a great success rate in managing it. Elbow pain can affect anyone who is involved in construction or sports. Elbow pain can also be related to arthritis, inflammation, sprains and bursitis and over-using the elbow in moving and bending is going to cause it to become inflamed and swell.

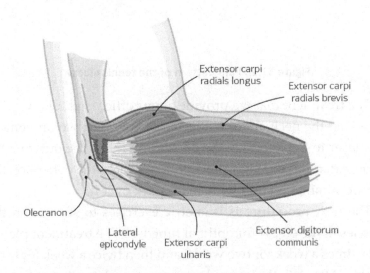

Figure 36. Example of Elbow pain due to overuse.

Tennis elbow affects the outer layer of tissue, however, the Golfer's Elbow is the inner aspect of the injured area. The pain does not go away on its own and using physical therapy isometric exercises and injecting cortisone does not provide a long lasting relieve. The pain will cause diminished productivity as well as decreased athletic performance.

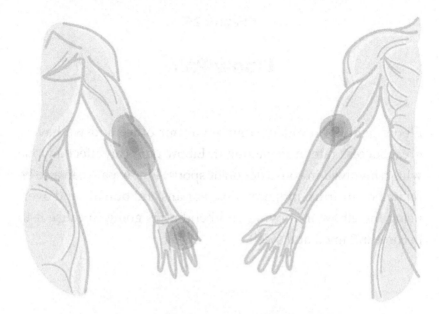

Figure 37.18 Pain pattern of the tennis elbow.

The treatment that we provide at our office is as follows: first we adjust the neck and the affected elbow, then we implement cold laser to the affected side depending if it is the outer or the inner. After the cold laser procedure, we place the patient on the electric stimulation unit with an ice pack over it.

The next procedure is isometric exercises to strengthen the muscles in the elbow for optimal function. The treatment plan is three times a week for two weeks and then twice a week for three weeks. After all the procedures are complete, the patient is wrapped with Kinesio tape and ordered to wear it for 24 hours (including taking a shower with it.)

The patient recovery varies with this condition, but we have seen 85% to 95% improvement which is much better than 70% or worse which is typically the average.

Chapter 27

Hip Pain

Hip pain carries a wide range of disorders that we see in our office. These conditions include arthritis, inflammation, overuse for compensating for low back pain, and degeneration. Most hip conditions we see are as a result of disc degeneration in the low back.

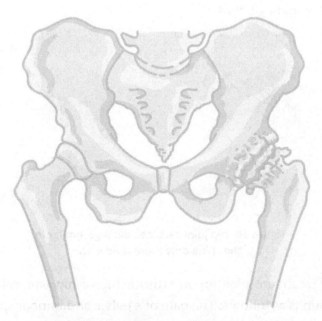

Figure 38. On the right you see the deformed hip joint called (mushroom hip).

As mentioned earlier, there are no patients that come and treat their pain as a first-occurring condition. They are typically going to wait until the last minute, and then make the final decision to do something about it. Therefore, a single episode of just hip pain we hardly ever see in our office. Sometimes the deformity of the hip is beyond conservative management and surgery is recommended.

The surgeries are 95% successful and the orthotic hip made of plastic lasts for twenty years. Also, the recovery rate is short, you do not need to stay at the hospital for a long time and can be release the following day. The reason for that is very simple. The hip has a very rich blood supply that delivers nutrients into the bone. Since most of our patients are Baby Boomers who do not like any kind of surgeries and are very proactive, they prefer conservative management.

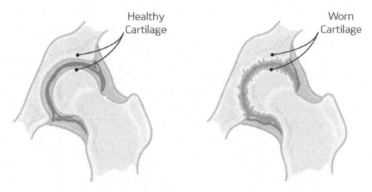

Healthy Cartilage

Worn Cartilage

Figure 39. Hip joint cartilage damage similar in the spine only there is no disc.

The treatment plan for an arthritic hip or hip pain related to back pain is as follows: The patient's pelvis and lumbar spine are adjusted first to clear out the compensatory pain. Then the hip is adjusted to remove any misalignments that caused the dysfunction from the get-go. Third, the cold laser is placed on the outer area of the hip to get the laser light inside the joint space for four minutes for the first intensive phase where it could be three times a week for three weeks or even prolonged plan for three times a week for four weeks. Then it drops down to three minutes twice a week. As the patient's pain diminishes, the cold laser treatment can be reduced to two minutes per procedure.

The next phase of care is functional rehab for strengthening the spine and all the muscles surrounding the hip; these include flexors, extensors, adductors, and abductors. If the pain is unbearable where the patient can't put any weight on it, we use Kinesio taping where the patient has bundles of tape placed on the buttock, the front of the leg, and across the hip, to eliminate the amount of pressure exerted by the patient.

The treatment protocol varies from three times a week for three to four weeks, with a gradual reduction to twice a week for three or four weeks. The success rate we see at our clinic with chronic arthritis hip pain is between 80 to 97%!

Chapter 28

Tolerance to Pain

This is a very personal and interesting topic for me as a practitioner and an athlete; but patients do not want to hear your war stories when it comes to teaching them about pain. When I was a kid, I never had time to listen to a doctor who did not practice what he preaches and was giving me advice to never work out because I was disabled due to injury.

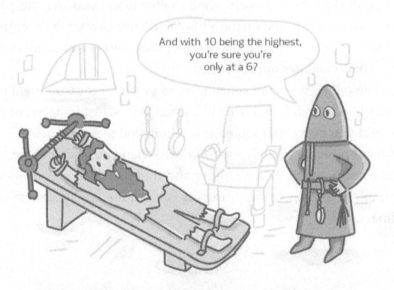

Figure 40. Again, Pain and Function are two different animals

Every patient is more concerned with function of the spine and not pain. The pain killers that are currently meant to diminish pain, do not address the function of the patient. Patients go in to see doctors not because of their pain, but inability or diminished quality of life. That is a fact. I have heard countless times, patients telling me that they have a high tolerance for pain, but that this time, the pain was unbearable.

Really it was?

You barely got out of the car and walked to my office, but the pain is unbearable? How many times do we have unspecified episodes of pain coming out everywhere from our body, but do we run to go see a doctor right away? The answer is no. Because we go see a doctor when we can't bend down or do the things we normally could do.

That is not a Chiropractic Theory it is a Universal Theory that is a common practice for every physician, whether it is Orthopedic Surgeon, Medical Doctor Physical Therapist, Massage Therapist or a Chiropractor. That is why there is a disability questionnaire in the office of every good doctor who measures the patient's outcome based on the ability to do things after their injury or self-developed condition. Each of these tests carry numerical data that validates improvement.

The pain level is not considered as much for measurement of pain, however, it is still used in United States. Just imagine, how would you prove that someone is telling you that their pain level is 8 out possible 10 in their shoulder? When you ask a patient to lift an object with their shoulder and they are unable to, or then complain of pain doing it, then it is considered a syndrome or illness.

Chapter 29

Maintenance Care

What is maintenance care? It is a treatment plan that is prescribed after you have had reached a maximum medical improvement from your illness or injury. An example of this would be someone who had chronic low back pain, numbness and tingling in their leg and was treated for certain number of visits. Then they got better, function has returned back to a normal quality of life and is back to pre-injury status.

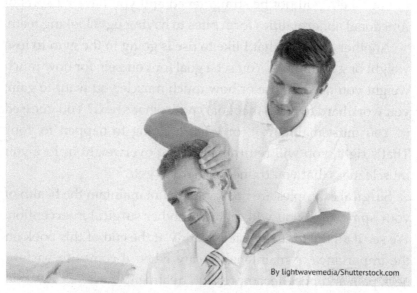

By lightwavemedia/Shutterstock.com

Figure 41. Maintenance care plans are starting to get recognized by the insurance companies.

At this point, maintenance care is recommended to maintain the results they have gained during their treatment plan. The plan is asymptomatic which means that the patient does not necessarily need to have muscle spasms, decreased range of motion or residual pain.

The maintenance plan is designed to preserve the health of your spine and to prevent any catastrophic flair-ups that can potentially return you back to how you were when you came in to see the Doctor. If you have been battling weight loss or were placed on protein diets, do you go back and eat anything you want at that point or you maintain a healthy diet for the rest of your life? I think you know the answer.

Dentists have been utilizing maintenance plans for years when they prescribe braces for your teeth. You have to wear braces for two years, then you have to wear the retainers for another three years and if you take them earlier than you supposed to your teeth will not be straightened and you have all sorts of functional abnormalities form bites to having ugly looking teeth.

Another example that I like to use is going to the gym to lose weight or gain muscle. You set a goal for yourself for how much weight you need to lose or how much muscle you want to gain; you work hard to reach that goal - now what's next? You guessed it! You must maintain it, or what is going to happen to you? That's right, you will return back being overweight or lose you muscle mass that you trained so hard to get.

Surgical examples are no. If you do not maintain the health of your spine, then you will require another surgical intervention. We see it all the time. I posted a study at the end of this book on the importance of maintenance care when it comes to back or neck pain and post decompression treatment.

Chapter 30

Reverse Cervical Curve

What is Reverse Cervical Curve? This is when your bones in your neck are curved the opposite way. For example, the bones in the spine of an average person look like the inverted letter "C" (please see the example below.)

While the spinal structure of a person with an abnormal curve will look like the actual letter "C". The patient would feel constant headaches with tearing of the eyes and severe neck pain. Due to the positioning of the curve, there is constant pressure on the spinal discs that put pressure on the nerves causing numbness and tingling in the arms and fingers.

Imagine someone actually bowed your spine and started pulling on it with their arms and feet at the same time. That would not feel very nice would it? So, the only way to change the structural foundation of the cervical spine, "neck bones," is to actually perform a cosmetic repair. I am not talking about changing the bones in the neck, I am talking about changing the letter "C" curve into the reverse letter "C" curve.

This particular protocol is very similar as the ones that have been mentioned earlier in this book concerning scoliosis. The patient is lying face down on the table, spinal manipulation of the neck is performed face down on the right; then if indicated, on the left side of the patient. The patient is instructed to perform homework exercises by placing a bunch of couch-like pillows under their upper back and lay on them for twenty minutes, five times a week while treating.

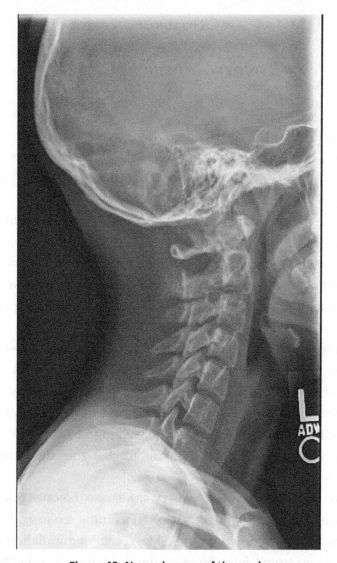

Figure 42. Normal curve of the neck.

The protocol depends on how much curvature the patient needs to achieve. If the goal is between a 15-20% curvature, then the patient can be seen three times a week for six weeks, and then gradually reduce to twice a week for six weeks.

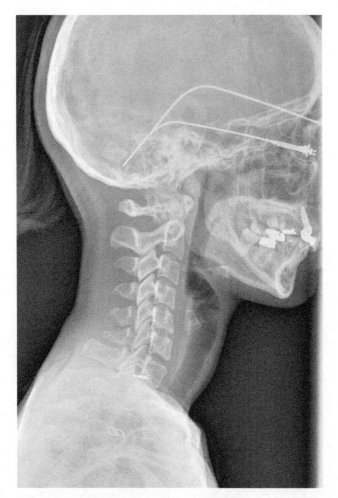

Figure 43. The picture on the right is abnormal curve of the neck that produces pain and headaches.

Functional rehab is necessary to reduce muscle tension from the inverted curve that pulls all of the anatomical structures in the opposite direction from how the body is supposed to normally function. This type of cosmetic protocol is far more favorable than the surgical intervention of placing rods to increase the angles of the neck and has a success rate among patients at 98%!

Chapter 31

Shoulder Girdle Instability

Shoulder girdle instability is related to the neck instability. When someone develops chronic neck pain, they are going to adopt a certain postural adaptability. One shoulder is going to be pulled down, while the other shoulder will be pulled up. If you or someone you know has had, or currently has, chronic neck pain have them stand against the wall and look at their neck and shoulder. You will see that their shoulder-line not level, and their head is tilted to the side. The reason for that is because the head is not sitting properly in respect to the shoulder girdle. When that person takes a deep breath and exhales you can see that their clavicle moves up and the other one doesn't.

The other confirmatory test would be to have the patient turn around and observe their scapula bones move up or down. In a person with a postural girdle misalignment, you will see that during inhalation and exhalation, the scapula on the same side on the clavicle does not move; in other words, if the patient's right clavicle did not move up as it should during breathing, the right scapula will not move either.

If the patient's neck is treated but the shoulder girdle is not supported properly then the treatment will not hold due the girdle pulling the muscles away and into the side of the immovable clavicle and scapula. It is like building a house without the foundation. If there is no foundation, then the house will collapse with structural damage, the same applies to the shoulder girdle that support the neck.

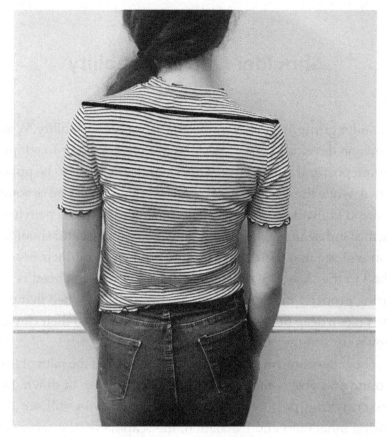

Figure 44. Uneven shoulders.

The protocol for correction of the girdle is to adjust the neck on the sides that are indicated during the analysis, then manipulate the scapula down and out and from straight up as the patient is laying down; then the patients turns over on their stomach and his scapula is adjusted straight up by aligning the shoulder girdle into a normal, horizontal position for the patient's neck and shoulders.

The post checkup can be performed by having the patient stand against the wall with an even line across their neck and shoulders. Also, upon inhalation and exhalation you can observe symmetrical movement of the clavicles and scapula.

The protocol can be repeated for several treatments, but I have not seen it being implemented more than three visits for a permanent hold. Pretty Amazing Stuff!

Chapter 32

Conclusion

As mentioned earlier medicine is not an exact science, and that is why you see that there was no standard100 % protocol that has healed every patient with certainty.

But what I can tell you with a high degree of reasonable probability, is that these spinal protocols are more than 96% effective in all of these disorders mentioned. If it was not for these protocols, there would no Dr. Alan Khiger who implements them daily for his patients and using it on himself to continue the love for the Martial Arts and weight training.

So, if you take the 88% of the current population who are suffering from chronic disease of neck and back pain, then there can be a lot of lives that can be saved each year from surgeries and getting rid of disabling pain that reduces productivity that destroys families.

No one can hurt you more than you can hurt yourself; whether it is through your mistakes in life or wrong decision making. But there is always success that is built from your failures. I highly recommend the movie "The Secret" for anyone to watch. In my 43 years of my life I have seen misery and happiness in health, business, and personal life. I preach daily to my patients and my staff that achieving a balance in life will come from you first. Only then you can inspire others by achieving greatness within yourself.

Once this book is published, it's going to spread like cancer (in a good way!) among people who are looking for the alternative health solutions that carry fact-based protocols tested on real patients and proven to work!

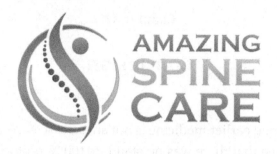

WEBSITE: www.AmazingSpineCare.com
EMAIL: amazingspinecare@gmail.com
PHONE: (904) 701-3916

Locations
South side:
6320 St. Augustine Rd. Ste.1
Jacksonville, FL 32217

Beach Blvd:
2907 Sping Glen Rd.,
Jacksonville, FL 32207

West Side:
5233 Ricker Rd. Ste. 102
Jacksonville, FL 32210

Orange Park:
1543 Kingsley Ave., Ste. 9

Jacksonville, FL, 32073
North Side:
3000 Dunn Ave, Ste. 13,
Jacksonville, FL 32218

APPENDIX – Research Articles

PLoS One. 2018 Sep 12;13(9):e0203029. doi: 10.1371/journal.pone.0203029. eCollection 2018.

The Nordic Maintenance Care program: Effectiveness of chiropractic maintenance care versus symptom-guided treatment for recurrent and persistent low back pain-A pragmatic randomized controlled trial.

Eklund A[1], Jensen I[1], Lohela-Karlsson M[1], Hagberg J[1], Leboeuf-Yde C[2], Kongsted A[3,4], Bodin L[1], Axén I[1,2].

Author information

1 Karolinska Institutet, Institute of Environmental Medicine, Unit of Intervention and Implementation Research for Worker Health, Stockholm, Sweden.
2 Institute for Regional Health Research, University of Southern Denmark, Odense, Denmark.
3 Nordic Institute of Chiropractic and Clinical Biomechanics, Odense, Denmark.
4 Department of Sports Science and Clinical Biomechanics, University of Southern Denmark, Odense, Denmark.

Abstract

BACKGROUND: For individuals with recurrent or persistent non-specific low back pain (LBP), exercise and exercise combined with education have been shown to be effective in preventing new episodes or in reducing the impact of the condition. Chiropractors have traditionally used Maintenance Care (MC), as secondary and tertiary prevention strategies. The aim of this trial was to investigate the effectiveness of MC on pain trajectories for patients with recurrent or persistent LBP.

METHOD: This pragmatic, investigator-blinded, two arm randomized controlled trial included consecutive patients (18-65 years old) with non-specific LBP, who had an early favorable response to chiropractic care. After an initial course of treatment, eligible subjects were randomized to either MC or control (symptom-guided treatment). The primary outcome was total number of days with bothersome LBP during 52 weeks collected weekly with text-messages (SMS) and estimated by a GEE model.

RESULTS: Three hundred and twenty-eight subjects were randomly allocated to one of the two treatment groups. MC resulted in a reduction in the total number of days per week with bothersome LBP compared with symptom-guided treatment. During the 12 month study period, the MC group (n = 163, 3 dropouts) reported 12.8 (95% CI = 10.1, 15.5; p = <0.001) fewer days in total with bothersome LBP compared to the control group (n = 158, 4 dropouts) and received 1.7 (95% CI = 1.8, 2.1; p = <0.001) more treatments. Numbers presented are means. No serious adverse events were recorded.

CONCLUSION: MC was more effective than symptom-guided treatment in reducing the total number of days over 52 weeks with bothersome non-specific LBP but it resulted in a higher number of treatments. For selected patients with recurrent or persistent non-specific LBP who respond well to an initial course of chiropractic care, MC should be considered an option for tertiary prevention.

PMID: 30208070

PMCID: PMC6135505

DOI: 10.1371/journal.pone.0203029
[Indexed for MEDLINE]

Free PMC Article

J Phys Ther Sci. 2017 Nov;29(11):2062-2067. doi: 10.1589/jpts.29.2062. Epub 2017 Nov 24.

Reduction of progressive thoracolumbar adolescent idiopathic scoliosis by chiropractic biophysics® (CBP®) mirror image® methods following failed traditional chiropractic treatment: a case report.

Haggard JS[1], Haggard JB[1], Oakley PA[2], Harrison DE[3].

Author information

1 Private Practice, USA.
2 Private Practice: 11A-1100 Gorham Street, Newmarket, ON, L3Y 8Y8, Canada.
3 CBP NonProfit, Inc., USA.

Abstract

[Purpose] To present a case demonstrating the reduction of progressive thoracolumbar scoliosis by incorporating Chiropractic BioPhysics® (CBP®) technique's mirror image® exercises, traction and blocking procedures based on the 'non-commutative properties of finite rotation angles under addition' engineering law. [Subject and Methods] A 15-year-old female presented with a right thoracolumbar scoliosis having a Cobb angle from T5-L3 of 27° and suffering from headaches and lower back pains. Her curve had progressed over the last two years despite being under traditional chiropractic care. [Results] The patient was treated using CBP structural rehabilitation protocols incorporating mirror image traction, home blocking, corrective exercises and spinal manipulation. The patient was treated 24 times (including 45 home self-treatment blocking sessions) over the course of 15-weeks. Her thoracolumbar curve reduced from 27° to 8° and her headache and low back pain disability improved significantly. [Conclusion] CBP mirror image exercises and traction are consistent with other successful non-surgical approaches and show promise in treating adolescent idiopathic scoliosis.

PMID: 29200657
PMCID:PMC5702847
DOI:10.1589/jpts.29.2062

Free PMC Article

Mechanical Traction for Lumbar Radicular Pain: Supine or Prone? A Randomized Controlled Trial.

BilgilisoyFiliz   M[1], Kiliç   Z, Uçkun   A, Çakir   T, KoldaşDoğan Ş, Toraman NF.

Author information

1 From the Antalya Training and Research Hospital, Department of Physical Medicine and Rehabilitation, Antalya, Turkey (MBF, ŞKD, NFT); Antalya Atatürk State Hospital, Physical Medicine and Rehabilitation Clinic, Antalya, Turkey (ZK); Mut State Hospital, Physical Medicine and Rehabilitation Clinic, Mersin, Turkey (AU); and Private Likya Hospital, Physical Medicine and Rehabilitation Clinic, Antalya, Turkey (TÇ).

Abstract

OBJECTIVE: The aim of the study was to compare the effects of mechanical lumbar traction either in the supine or in the prone position with conventional physical therapy (PT) in patients with chronic low back pain and lumbosacral nerve root involvement in terms of disability, pain, and mobility.

DESIGN: Participants (N = 125) were randomly assigned to receive 15 sessions of PT with additional mechanical lumbar traction either in the supine position (supine traction group) or in the prone position (prone traction group) or only PT without traction (PT only group). Patients were assessed at baseline and at the end of the PT sessions in terms of disability, pain, and mobility. Disability was assessed using the modified Oswesty Disability Index; pain was assessed using a visual analog scale, and lumbar mobility was assessed using the modified lumbar Schober test.

RESULTS: One hundred eighteen patients completed the trial. All groups improved significantly in the Oswesty Disability Index, visual analog scale, and modified lumbar Schober test ($P < 0.05$). In the between-group analysis, improvements of Oswesty Disability Index and visual analog scale were found significantly better in the prone traction group compared with the PT only group (adjusted $P = 0.031$ and 0.006, respectively).

CONCLUSIONS: Addition of traction in the prone position to other modalities resulted in larger immediate improvements in terms of pain and disability, and the results suggest that when using traction, prone traction might be first choice. Further research is needed to confirm the benefits of lumbar traction in the prone position.

Chiropr Man Therap. 2019 Feb 5;27:6. doi: 10.1186/s12998-018-0225-8. eCollection 2019.

An observational study on trajectories and outcomes of chronic low back pain patients referred from a spine surgery division for chiropractic treatment.

Wirth B[1], Riner F[1], Peterson C[1], Humphreys BK[1], Farshad M[2], Becker S[3], Schweinhardt P[1].

Author information

1 Integrative Spinal Research Group, Department of Chiropractic Medicine, Balgrist University Hospital, Forchstr. 340, 8008 Zurich, Switzerland.
2 Spine Division, Department of Orthopedics, Balgrist University Hospital, Zurich, Switzerland.
3 Department of Cognitive and Clinical Neuroscience, Central Institute of Mental Health, Medical Faculty Mannheim, Heidelberg University, Mannheim, Germany.

Abstract

BACKGROUND: A close collaboration between surgeons and non-surgical spine experts is crucial for optimal care of low back pain (LBP) patients. The affiliation of a chiropractic teaching clinic to a university hospital with a large spine division in Zurich, Switzerland, enables such collaboration. The aim of this study was to describe the trajectories and outcomes of patients with chronic LBP referred from the spine surgery division to the chiropractic teaching clinic.

METHODS: The patients filled in an 11-point numeric rating scale (NRS) for pain intensity and the Bournemouth Questionnaire (BQ) (bio-psycho-social measure) at baseline and after

1 week, 1, 3, 6 and 12 months. Additionally, the Patient's Global Impression of Change (PGIC) scale was recorded at all time points apart from baseline. The courses of NRS and BQ were analyzed using linear mixed model analysis and repeated measures ANOVA. The proportion of patients reporting clinically relevant overall improvement (PGIC) was calculated and the underlying factors were determined using logistic regression analyses.

RESULTS: Between June 2014 and October 2016, 67 participants (31 male, mean age = 46.8 ± 17.6 years) were recruited, of whom 46 had suffered from LBP for > 1 year, the rest for > 3 months, but < 1 year. At baseline, mean NRS was 5.43 (SD 2.37) and mean BQ was 39.80 (SD 15.16) points. NRS significantly decreased [F(5, 106.77) = 3.15, p = 0.011] to 4.05 (SD 2.88) after 12 months. A significant reduction was not observed before 6 months after treatment start (p = 0.04). BQ significantly diminished [F(5, 106.47) = 6.55, p < 0.001] to 29.00 (SD 17.96) after 12 months and showed a significant reduction within the first month (p < 0.01). The proportion of patients reporting overall improvement significantly increased from 23% after 1 week to 47% after 1 month (p = 0.004), when it stabilized [56% after 3 and 6 months, 44% after 12 months]. Reduction in bio-psycho-social impairment (BQ) was of higher importance for overall improvement than pain reduction.

CONCLUSIONS: Chiropractic treatment is a valuable conservative treatment modality associated with clinically relevant improvement in approximately half of patients with chronic LBP. These findings provide an example of the importance of interdisciplinary collaboration in the treatment of chronic back pain patients.

Spine (Phila Pa 1976). 2019 May 1;44(9):647-651. doi: 10.1097/BRS.0000000000002902.

Group and Individual-level Change on Health-related Quality of Life in Chiropractic Patients With Chronic Low Back or Neck Pain.

Hays RD[1], Spritzer KL[1], Sherbourne CD[2], Ryan GW[2], Coulter ID[3].

Author information

1 Division of General Internal Medicine & Health Services Research, UCLA Department of Medicine, Los Angeles, CA.
2 RAND Health, Santa Monica, CA.
3 UCLA School of Dentistry, Los Angeles, CA.

Abstract

STUDY DESIGN: A prospective observational study.

OBJECTIVE: The aim of this study was to evaluate group-level and individual-level change in health-related quality of life among persons with chronic low back pain or neck pain receiving chiropractic care in the United States.

SUMMARY OF BACKGROUND DATA: Chiropractors treat chronic low back and neck pain, but there is limited evidence of the effectiveness of their treatment METHODS.: A 3-month longitudinal study of 2024 patients with chronic low back pain or neck pain receiving care from 125 chiropractic clinics at six locations throughout the United States was conducted. Ninety-one percent of the sample completed the baseline and 3-month follow-up survey (n=1835). Average age was 49, 74% females, and most of the sample had a college degree, were non-Hispanic

White, worked full-time, and had an annual income of $60,000 or more. Group-level (within-group t tests) and individual-level (coefficient of repeatability) changes on the Patient-Reported Outcomes Measurement Information System (PROMIS-29) v2.0 profile measure was evaluated: six multi-item scales (physical functioning, pain, fatigue, sleep disturbance, social health, emotional distress) and physical and mental health summary scores.

RESULTS: Within-group t tests indicated significant group-level change (P<0.05) for all scores except for emotional distress, and these changes represented small improvements in health (absolute value of effect sizes ranged from 0.08 for physical functioning to 0.20 for pain). From 13% (physical functioning) to 30% (PROMIS-29 v2.0 Mental Health Summary Score) got better from baseline to 3 months later according to the coefficient of repeatability.

CONCLUSION: Chiropractic care was associated with significant group-level improvement in health-related quality of life over time, especially in pain. But only a minority of the individuals in the sample got significantly better ("responders"). This study suggests some benefits of chiropractic on functioning and well-being of patients with low back pain or neck pain.

J Manipulative PhysiolTher. 2015 Sep;38(7):477-83. doi: 10.1016/j.jmpt.2015.06.015. Epub 2015 Aug 16.
First-contact care with a medical vs chiropractic provider after consultation with a swiss telemedicine provider: comparison of outcomes, patient satisfaction, and health care costs in spinal, hip, and shoulder pain patients.

Houweling TA[1], Braga AV[2], Hausheer T[3], Vogelsang M[4], Peterson C[5], Humphreys BK[6].

Author information

1 Postdoctoral Research Fellow, Department of Chiropractic Medicine, University Hospital Balgrist, Forchstrasse 340, 8008 Zürich, Switzerland. Electronic address: taco.houweling@balgrist.ch.
2 CEO and Founder, bragamed GmbH, Baar, Switzerland.
3 Clinician, Private Practice, Wädenswil, Switzerland.
4 Clinician, Private Practice, Zürich, Switzerland.
5 Professor, Department of Chiropractic Medicine, University Hospital Balgrist, Zürich, Switzerland.
6 Professor and Head of Department, Department of Chiropractic Medicine, University Hospital Balgrist, Zürich, Switzerland.

Abstract

OBJECTIVE: The purpose of this study was to identify differences in outcomes, patient satisfaction, and related health care costs in spinal, hip, and shoulder pain patients who initiated care with medical doctors (MDs) vs those who initiated care with doctors of chiropractic (DCs) in Switzerland.

METHODS: A retrospective double cohort design was used. A self-administered questionnaire was completed by first-contact care spinal, hip, and shoulder pain patients who, 4 months previously, contacted a Swiss telemedicine provider regarding advice about their complaint. Related health care costs were determined in a subsample of patients by reviewing the claims database of a Swiss insurance provider.

RESULTS: The study sample included 403 patients who had seen MDs and 316 patients who had seen DCs as initial health care providers for their complaint. Differences in patient sociodemographic characteristics were found in terms of age, pain location, and mode of onset. Patients initially consulting MDs had significantly less reduction in their numerical pain rating score (difference of 0.32) and were significantly less likely to be satisfied with the care received (odds ratio = 1.79) and the outcome of care (odds ratio = 1.52). No significant differences were found for Patient's Global Impression of Change ratings. Mean costs per patient over 4 months were significantly lower in patients initially consulting DCs (difference of CHF 368; US $368).

CONCLUSION: Spinal, hip, and shoulder pain patients had clinically similar pain relief, greater satisfaction levels, and lower overall cost if they initiated care with DCs, when compared with those who initiated care with MDs.

J Altern Complement Med. 2019 Aug 27. doi: 10.1089/acm.2019.0247. [Epub ahead of print]

Prevalence and Characteristics of Chronic Spinal Pain Patients with Different Hopes (TreatmentGoals) for Ongoing Chiropractic Care.

Herman PM[1], Edgington SE[1], Ryan GW[1], Coulter ID[1].

Author information

1 RAND Corporation, Santa Monica, CA.

Abstract

Objectives: The treatment goals of patients successfully using ongoing provider-based care for chronic spinal pain can help inform health policy related to this care.

Design: Multinomial logistical hierarchical linear models were used to examine the characteristics of patients with different treatment goals for their ongoing care.

Settings/Location: Observational data from a large national sample of patients from 125 chiropractic clinics clustered in 6 U.S. regions.

Subjects: Patients with nonwork-injury-related nonspecific chronic low-back pain (CLBP) and chronic neck pain (CNP).

Interventions: All were receiving ongoing chiropractic care.

Outcome measures: Primary outcomes were patient endorsement of one of four goals for their treatment. Explanatory variables included pain characteristics, pain beliefs, goals for mobility/flexibility, demographics, and other psychological variables.

Results: Across our sample of 1614 patients (885 with CLBP and 729 with CNP) just under one-third endorsed a treatment goal of having their pain go away permanently (cure). The rest had goals of preventing their pain from coming back (22% CLBP, 16% CNP); preventing their pain from getting worse (14% CLBP, 12% CNP); or temporarily relieving their pain (31% CLBP, 41% CNP). In univariate analysis across these goals, patients differed significantly on almost all variables. In the multinomial logistic models, a goal of cure was associated with shorter pain duration and more belief in a medical cure; a goal of preventing pain from coming back was associated with lower pain levels; and those with goals of preventing their pain from getting worse or temporarily relieving pain were similar, including in having their pain longer.

Conclusions: Although much of health policy follows a curative model, the majority of these CLBP and CNP patients have goals of pain management (using ongoing care) rather than "cure" (care with a specific end) for their chiropractic care. This information could be useful in crafting policy for patients facing provider-based nonpharmacologic care for chronic pain.

Efficacy of spinal manipulation for chronic headache: a systematic review.

Bronfort G[1], Assendelft WJ, Evans R, Haas M, Bouter L.

Author information

1 Department of Research, Wolfe-Harris Center for Clinical Studies, Northwestern Health Sciences University, Bloomington, MN 55431, USA. gbronfort@nwhealth.edu

Abstract

BACKGROUND: Chronic headache is a prevalent condition with substantial socioeconomic impact. Complementary or alternative therapies are increasingly being used by patients to treat headache pain, and spinal manipulative therapy (SMT) is among the most common of these.

OBJECTIVE: To assess the efficacy/effectiveness of SMT for chronic headache through a systematic review of randomized clinical trials.

STUDY SELECTION: Randomized clinical trials on chronic headache (tension, migraine and cervicogenic) were included in the review if they compared SMT with other interventions or placebo. The trials had to have at least 1 patient-rated outcome measure such as pain severity, frequency, duration, improvement, use of analgesics, disability, or quality of life. Studies were identified through a comprehensive search of MEDLINE (1966-1998) and EMBASE (1974-1998). Additionally, all available data from the Cumulative Index of Nursing and Allied Health Literature, the Chiropractic Research Archives Collection, and the Manual, Alternative, and Natural Therapies Information System were used, as well as material gathered through the citation tracking, and hand searching of non-indexed chiropractic, osteopathic, and manual medicine journals.

DATA EXTRACTION: Information about outcome measures, interventions and effect sizes was used to evaluate treatment efficacy. Levels of evidence were determined by a classification system incorporating study validity and statistical significance of study results. Two authors independently extracted data and performed methodological scoring of selected trials.

Nine trials involving 683 patients with chronic headache were included. The methodological quality (validity) scores ranged from 21 to 87 (100-point scale). The trials were too heterogeneous in terms of patient clinical characteristic, control groups, and outcome measures to warrant statistical pooling. Based on predefined criteria, there is moderate evidence that SMT has short-term efficacy similar to amitriptyline in the prophylactic treatment of chronic tension-type headache and migraine. SMT does not appear to improve outcomes when added to soft-tissue massage for episodic tension-type headache. There is moderate evidence that SMT is more efficacious than massage for cervicogenic headache. Sensitivity analyses showed that the results and the overall study conclusions remained the same even when substantial changes in the prespecified assumptions/rules regarding the evidence determination were applied.

CONCLUSIONS: SMT appears to have a better effect than massage for cervicogenic headache. It also appears that SMT has an effect comparable to commonly used first-line prophylactic prescription medications for tension-type headache and migraine headache. This conclusion rests upon a few trials of adequate methodological quality. Before any firm conclusions can be drawn, further testing should be done in rigorously designed, executed, and analyzed trials with follow-up periods of sufficient length.

Effects of Integrated Yoga Intervention on Psychopathologies and Sleep Quality Among Professional Caregivers of Older Adults With Alzheimer's Disease: A Controlled Pilot Study.

Chhugani KJ, Metri K, Babu N, Nagendra HR.

Abstract

CONTEXT: Providing care to patients suffering from chronic neurological problems is a stressful job. While providing care to the patients, professional caregivers experience various kinds of physical and mental challenges that affect their mental health and sleep. Yoga is a form of mind-body medicine shown to be an effective intervention in improving physical and mental health.

OBJECTIVE: To examine the effects of an integrated yoga (IY) intervention on anxiety, depression, stress, and sleep quality among professional caregivers of older adults with Alzheimer's disease.

SETTING: This study was conducted in an Alzheimer care institution located in Bangalore City in southern India.

PARTICIPANTS: Participants were professional female caregivers of older adults with Alzheimer's disease. Participant age range was between 20 and 50 y (mean, 34 ± 8.4 y). A total of 30 participants were enrolled in the study. Seventeen participants followed IY intervention and 13 were considered in a wait-list group.

INTERVENTION: Participants in the IY group received a structured IY intervention comprising yoga asanas, pranayama, meditation, and relaxation techniques, 1 h/d, 6 d/wk, for 1 mo. Participants in the wait-list control group followed their daily activities.

OUTCOME MEASURES: Blood pressure, heart rate, anxiety, depression, stress, and sleep quality were assessed at baseline after 1 mo for both the groups. Data were analyzed with an appropriate statistical test using SPSS Version 16 software (IBM, Armonk, NY, USA).

RESULTS: The IY group showed significant improvement in heart rate, blood pressure, stress, depression, anxiety, and sleep quality after 1 mo compared with baseline. In contrast to the IY group, the wait-listed control group showed significant increase in anxiety, depression, and stress and significant decrease in sleep quality after 1 mo compared with baseline.

CONCLUSIONS: The present study showed the potential use of IY intervention in reducing stress, anxiety, and depression. The study also suggests that IY improves sleep quality among professional caregivers. However, further studies using a randomized controlled trial method with a larger sample size and for a longer duration should be conducted to confirm the present findings.

Use of a multimodal conservative management protocol for the treatment of a patient with cervical radiculopathy.

Radpasand M.

Abstract

OBJECTIVE: The purpose of this study is to describe and discuss the treatment of a cervical disk herniation using a sequential multimodal conservative management approach.

CLINICAL FEATURES: A 40-year-old man had complaints of headache and severe sharp neck pain radiating to his left shoulder down to his arm, forearm, and hand. Results of electromyography/nerve conduction studies were abnormal. Magnetic resonance imaging revealed a large disk protrusion at C5-C6 with indentation of the thecal sac and a spur at the posterior margin. Moderate left neural foraminal narrowing was present at C5-C6 with narrowed intervertebral disk space at C5-C6 and C6-C7.

INTERVENTION AND OUTCOME: High-velocity, low-amplitude chiropractic manipulation; electrotherapy; ice; and exercise were used for treatment. The Neck Disability Index was used as a primary and electromyography/nerve conduction studies as a secondary outcome measurement. Based on the Neck Disability Index, there was an overall 89.65% symptoms improvement from the baseline.

CONCLUSIONS: This case study demonstrated possible beneficial effects of the multimodal treatment approach in a patient with cervical radiculopathy.

Movement and manual therapy for adults with arthritis: 2012 National Health Interview Survey.

Pure E[1], Terhorst L[2], Baker N[2].

Author information

1 University of Pittsburgh, Department of Occupational therapy, 4028 Forbes Tower, Pittsburgh, PA 15260, United States. Electronic address: Elise.Pure@gmail.com.
2 University of Pittsburgh, Department of Occupational therapy, 4028 Forbes Tower, Pittsburgh, PA 15260, United States.

Abstract

BACKGROUND: The use of manual therapies (chiropractic manipulation, massage) and movement therapies (yoga, tai chi) by people with arthritis may relate to their personal characteristics, and the reported emotional and physical health outcomes may differ by type of therapy.

OBJECTIVES: To describe personal characteristics and predictors of manual and movement therapy use for people with arthritis, and to compare the use of manual versus movement therapy to improve physical and emotional health outcomes for people with arthritis.

METHODOLOGY: CAM respondents with arthritis were identified from the 2012 National Health Interview Survey (n = 8229). Data were analyzed to determine the overall percentages of CAM users, and to examine the associations between use/nonuse using multivariable linear regressions.

RESULTS: White, well-educated, physically active females were more likely to use both types of therapy. Movement therapy users reported positive emotional health outcomes twice as much as manual therapy users and 10% more reported positive physical health outcomes.

CONCLUSION: While both movement and manual therapies can have positive effects on people with arthritis, it appears that active therapies are more beneficial than passive therapies.

Are non-invasive interventions effective for the management of headaches associated with neck pain? An update of the Bone and Joint Decade Task Force on Neck Pain and Its Associated Disorders by the Ontario Protocol for Traffic Injury Management (OPTIMa) Collaboration.

PURPOSE: To update findings of the 2000-2010 Bone and Joint Decade Task Force on Neck Pain and its Associated Disorders and evaluate the effectiveness of non-invasive and non-pharmacological interventions for the management of patients with headaches associated with neck pain (i.e., tension-type, cervicogenic, or whiplash-related headaches).

METHODS: We searched five databases from 1990 to 2015 for randomized controlled trials (RCTs), cohort studies, and case-control studies comparing non-invasive interventions with other interventions, placebo/sham, or no interventions. Random pairs of independent reviewers critically appraised eligible studies using the Scottish Intercollegiate Guidelines Network criteria to determine scientific admissibility. Studies with a low risk of bias were synthesized following best evidence synthesis principles.

RESULTS: We screened 17,236 citations, 15 studies were relevant, and 10 had a low risk of bias. The evidence suggests that episodic tension-type headaches should be managed with low load endurance craniocervical and cervicoscapular exercises. Patients with chronic tension-type headaches may also benefit from low load endurance craniocervical and cervicoscapular exercises; relaxation training with stress coping therapy; or multimodal care that includes spinal mobilization, craniocervical exercises, and postural correction. For cervicogenic headaches, low load endurance craniocervical and cervicoscapular exercises; or manual therapy (manipulation with or without mobilization) to the cervical and thoracic spine may also be helpful.

CONCLUSIONS: The management of headaches associated with neck pain should include exercise. Patients who suffer from chronic tension-type headaches may also benefit from relaxation training with stress coping therapy or multimodal care. Patients with cervicogenic headache may also benefit from a course of manual therapy.

Review of Literature on Low-level Laser Therapy Benefits for Nonpharmacological Pain Control in Chronic Pain and Osteoarthritis.

Dima R, TieppoFrancio V, Towery C, Davani S.

Abstract

INTRODUCTION: Low-level laser therapy (LLLT) is a form of light therapy that triggers biochemical changes within cells. Photons are absorbed by cellular photoreceptors, triggering chemical alterations and potential biochemical benefits to the human body. LLLT has been used in pain management for years and is also known as cold laser therapy, which uses low-frequency continuous laser of typically 600 to 1000 nm wavelength for pain reduction and healing stimulation. Many studies have demonstrated analgesic and anti-inflammatory effects provided by photobiomodulation in both experimental and clinical trials.

OBJECTIVE: The purpose of this research article was to present a summary of the possible pain management benefits of LLLT.

RESULTS: In cold laser therapy, coherent light of wavelength 600 to 1000 nm is applied to an area of concern with hope for photo-stimulating the tissues in a way that promotes and accelerates healing. This is evidenced by the similarity in absorption spectra between oxidized cytochrome c oxidase and action spectra from biological responses to light. LLLT, using the properties of coherent light, has been seen to produce pain relief and fibroblastic regeneration in clinical trials and laboratory experiments. LLLT has also been seen to significantly reduce pain in the acute setting; it is proposed that LLLT is able to reduce pain by lowering the level of biochemical markers and oxidative stress, and the formation of edema and hemorrhage. Many studies have demonstrated analgesic and anti-inflammatory effects provided by photobiomodulation in both experimental and clinical trials.

CONCLUSION: Based on current research, the utilization of LLLT for pain management and osteoarthritic conditions may be a complementary strategy used in clinical practice to provide symptom management for patients suffering from osteoarthritis and chronic pain.

Made in the USA
Middletown, DE
30 August 2024

59743629R00076